As if by MAGIC

TRUE STORIES OF ORDINARY PEOPLE LIVING INTUITIVELY TO ACHIEVE THE IMPOSSIBLE

LUCY KOBIER

Along with 8 inspiring authors

ISBN: 978-1-964619-92-7

TABLE OF CONTENTS

INTRODUCTION

Welcome to *As If by Magic*, a collection of stories that celebrates the profound impact of intuition on our lives. This book brings together a diverse group of individuals who have embraced their inner wisdom and harnessed the power of intuition to create transformative change. Each narrative reflects the courage and discovery that comes from listening to one's inner voice and following a path of authenticity.

At its core, *As If by Magic* is a powerful reminder that our deepest insights and most authentic paths come from within. Intuition—the ability to understand or know something without the need for conscious reasoning—is a natural talent available to all of us. It is the quiet voice that nudges us in the right direction, the subtle feeling that reveals our true desires, and the inner wisdom that aligns us with our highest potential.

As If by Magic demonstrates how living intuitively can lead to profound personal transformation and success. The stories shared here showcase the real-world applications of intuition, offering insights into how embracing this inner guidance can unlock new possibilities, create meaningful change and find deeper fulfilment from within.

As If by Magic isn't just a book; it's an invitation to explore the potential of your own intuitive abilities. Through the experiences of the authors, you are encouraged to listen to your inner wisdom, trust your instincts, and take bold steps towards your true desires.

These are the stories of ordinary people who have harnessed the power of intuition to achieve extraordinary outcomes. By sharing their journeys, they aim to inspire you and encourage you to connect with your own inner guidance and embrace the magic that intuition can bring to your life.

The influence of William Whitecloud and his Natural Success methodology has guided many of our authors on their journey towards discovering and embracing their intuitive potential. His teachings have been a source of education, inspiration and empowerment for those who have contributed to this collection.

Thank you for joining us on this journey. We hope that these stories inspire you to tap into your own intuitive wisdom and discover the magic that lies within.

Trust your inner voice, step into the unknown and watch the extraordinary unfold—*As if by magic...*

With love and magic,
Lucy Kobier

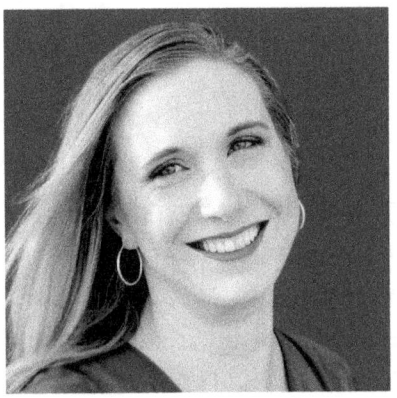

Lucy Kobier

Founder of Quantum Wellbeing

https://www.facebook.com/lucy.kobier/
https://www.lucykobier.com.au/home

Lucy Kobier is a visionary leader in holistic well-being and self-care, dedicated to empowering individuals to live authentically and intuitively. With a background in theology and personal development, Lucy has spent years exploring the intersection of faith and intuition, guiding others to discover their inner power and purpose. Her journey from overcoming personal challenges to embracing a life aligned with her true self serves as an inspiration to many. Through her work, Lucy helps people peel away layers of doubt and fear to uncover the clarity and fulfilment that lie within. She offers courses, workshops, and resources designed to support transformative growth. Lucy's passion for integrating science, spirituality, and personal empowerment shines through in everything she does, making her a sought-after mentor and speaker in the field of personal transformation.

Embracing Intuition and Finding Clarity

By Lucy Kobier

I don't think anyone considers their childhood idyllic. No matter how much time has passed, most of us can recall the moments that made our childhood feel less than perfect. We carry with us memories of feeling misunderstood, overlooked, or hurt, and those memories often shape how we see ourselves and the world around us. We tend to remember our childhoods not as a golden age of innocence, but as a series of experiences that, for better or worse (usually worse), left lasting impressions.

Even now, as I watch my own children grow, I notice something that both surprises and saddens me: They seem to latch onto the negative moments more strongly than the positive ones. Despite the love, support, and opportunities I try to provide them, it's the small, fleeting instances of disappointment or frustration that seem to stick with them the most. They're quick to form beliefs about themselves and the world. It's as if the good moments, no matter how plentiful, don't hook nearly as quickly or as deeply. Perhaps, it's just human nature, an instinct to protect ourselves by remembering the things that hurt us to avoid the same pain in the future.

I grew up in a large family as the sixth child of eight. Though I know it wasn't intentional, I often felt overlooked and insignificant—I felt invisible. It wasn't just the sheer number of siblings that made me feel this way; it was the quiet realization that, in a world where everyone else seemed to be seen and heard, I was somehow left in the background. My thoughts, my feelings, my very presence seemed to blend into the noise of the household, as if I were just another blurred shape in the crowd.

This feeling of invisibility was compounded by the fact that I was born with congenital cataracts. To the same degree that I felt unseen, nothing was truly visible to me either. My world was a perpetual blur, with faces and objects existing just beyond the edge of clarity. I knew there was a world beyond the fog I lived in—a world filled with colour, brightness, detail, and sharpness—but it was always just out of reach. I could sense it, I could feel it, but the only time I could truly see it was when I closed my eyes and imagined.

One of my early memories is of playing with my dad as a small child. He would shut his eyes, smiling, and say, "I can't see you, so you can't see me." At the time, it was just a game, a playful interaction meant to bring laughter, which it did. But as I grew older, I began to realize how much I had internalized this notion. In my mind, if I couldn't see the world clearly, then surely the world couldn't see me either. I was just a blur, a vague shape moving through life, much like how I experienced everything around me due to my cataracts.

The physical blur of my vision became a metaphor for my existence. I moved through my days with the same sense of detachment, as if the edges of my reality were always soft, always indistinct. I was present, but not fully seen—neither by others nor by myself. I knew there was more out there, a clearer, more vibrant life just beyond my reach, but it felt as though I were separated from it by a veil that I couldn't quite pierce.

It's only in my adult years that I've come to understand how deeply this belief took root in me. The idea that I was invisible because I couldn't see—that I was somehow less real, less important because my vision was impaired—shaped so much of how I interacted with the world. It wasn't just that I felt invisible in a large family; it was that I genuinely believed my lack of sight meant a lack of presence. I was as much a blur to others as the world was to me.

Through my childhood and teen years, 'coke bottle' glasses corrected my vision enough to help me with near-sighted things, but I was still quite visually impaired when it came to focusing on anything more than a meter or so away from me. I remember avoiding meeting friends in the shopping centre as a teenager because I could never recognize them from a distance and often walked up to the wrong group of girls. Catching the bus, my main way of getting around, was always embarrassing. To have any hope of reading the bus number, I had to flag down every bus that went by my stop. This meant flagging the wrong buses, which the bus drivers never appreciated, and neither did I. When I was feeling shy or particularly self-conscious, I wouldn't flag down a bus, thinking it wasn't mine, only to realize it was as it zoomed past and the familiar sinking feeling in my stomach—I had just missed my bus.

There was a whole world happening around me. I was aware of it, I knew it was there, but no matter what I did—how thick my glasses were, how many reps I did of my eye exercises, or how many countless hours I spent with one or the other eye patched—I just couldn't see what I knew had to be there. I experienced brief moments of clarity when the lighting was just right, and something was right in front of me, but beyond that, I was quite blind.

My journey to discovering my intuition and the power it holds wasn't dissimilar to my experience growing up with cataract blindness. Just as the world around me remained a blur despite my thick glasses, so too did my life's purpose and direction remain unclear despite my best efforts. I knew there was more beyond my experience of life. I could sense it—a sixth sense—that there was more, that I was meant for more. I would catch glimpses of it, things would fall into focus for just a moment, just like when the lighting was just right, and it was right in front of me. But as quickly as the clarity came, it dissolved into a blur again, and I was never really able to focus on it, always just beyond my field of perception.

As I transitioned from childhood into adulthood, the challenges I faced evolved, but the underlying sense of invisibility and searching for clarity remained. My journey through adulthood reads very similarly to a lot of other people. Finish school, take a gap year (in my case, two), go to university, fall in love, have my heart broken by my first serious boyfriend, get a job, fall in love again, get married, buy a house, have babies... so far, so good. I was ticking all the boxes I knew were on the 'Society's To-Do List' for life. But why wasn't I feeling satisfied? Why wasn't I feeling fulfilled? I knew there was a life out there, full of colour, excitement, and joy, but from where I was sitting, it was blurry. Now and then, I would do something that brought me joy, and things near to me became clearer—like the day I held each of my children for the first time, getting a promotion at work, or winning a National Title in competitive cheerleading. In these moments, the people and events became clear, like putting on a pair of glasses. But beyond these moments, in the space in between, everything was blurry. What had I missed? Watching friends and family moving around me, all seeming like they had it figured out. I felt like I was treading water, not really sure which direction I was going in, or if I was moving at all. Throughout this whole time, I knew there was more. I got glimpses of it every now and then, but I still didn't know how to have it for myself.

I had grown up attending church regularly and even studied theology, but by the time I hit my mid-twenties, the questions I was asking couldn't be answered. The opinions I had and the manner I expressed them as a young, curious woman didn't go down very well with the middle-aged white men in leadership in my congregation, so it was suggested I might like to attend somewhere new. I attended a few different churches and still couldn't   find what I was looking for. So, I stopped going.

The shift in identity after becoming a mother was a harder transition than I had expected. I loved my baby girl more than the world itself, but in loving her, I lost myself. I no longer saw myself as successful in my career; I was a Mum. I was no longer competing in a sport I loved; I was a Mum. I loved my baby girl, and 21 months later, my son, but there was still this knowing inside that there had to be more. I knew there had to be another way—I just couldn't see it.

After the birth of my second child, things felt like they went from bad to worse. By this time, I had   lost my dad to cancer, and we had sold our family home. We were under financial stress, we were under baby and toddler stress, sleep-deprived, and not coping. Cracks started to show in my marriage. My marriage ended before my son turned one, and divorce followed. I was left to navigate the challenges of single parenting and depression alone. All the while, I was juggling high-pressure corporate roles that only added to my stress, and a run of failed relationships left me with heartache. Each failure, each heartbreak, each setback chipped away at my sense of self-worth. Like so many others in similar situations, I found myself questioning if I was doing enough, if I was enough. Without knowing how I even ended up here, I knew there had to be more to this thing called life than the miserable existence I had found myself fighting to just barely survive.

I threw myself into personal development, trying every modality I could find. I felt broken and needed to know how to fix myself   . I went deep down the rabbit holes of spirituality, neuroscience, and psychology. I devoured work from Jack Canfield, Dr. Caroline Dweck, and Dr. Joe Dispenza. Bits and pieces started to resonate, and taking the pieces that resonated, I started to apply them to my life, taking personal responsibility, focusing on what I wanted to create, and taking obvious actions.

It's interesting how we often associate our intuition with warning us about potential dangers or guiding us away from negative outcomes. That gut feeling that something isn't right, urging us to take or avoid a certain action. Yet, when it comes to positive outcomes, we rarely give our intuition the same credit. Instead, we might chalk it up to luck or coincidence, overlooking the role our intuition played in guiding us towards those successes.

Things started to change. Things were starting to fall into place, but I still didn't realize the small nudges and moments of clarity in the midst of the turmoil as intuition. But it was there—perhaps you have felt it too? The subtle feeling that despite the external noise, there is an inner voice calling you towards a better path. And perhaps, like me, you resisted it. Too stubborn and committed to perpetuating the living hell of barely surviving that I had created to pay it much attention. Yet, amid the chaos, there was a persistent whisper within me, a small but unwavering voice that said, "There is more to life than this." This voice, this intuition, was my beacon. It was a sense of purpose that I couldn't quite articulate but felt deeply and continued to pursue. It was as if I knew there was a greater vision for my life, even if I couldn't see it clearly yet. I now understand that this inner voice is a universal gift, accessible to everyone, regardless of their circumstances.

In 2020, I was introduced to William Whitecloud, and his work finally gave structure and clarity to what I had known had been there all along. Intuition is an inherent ability that exists within every individual, much like other natural senses. People from all walks of life, regardless of their background, have the capacity to tap into their intuition. This innate guidance system helps us make decisions, understand situations, and gain insights without the need for conscious reasoning.

Thankfully, the year I turned 18, my specialist said my eyes had stabilized enough to undergo the required surgery to remove my clouded cataract lenses and insert artificial lenses. Due to the nature of surgery on and around the eyes, the medical preference was to do the surgery under a local anaesthetic, rather than knocking me out cold with a general. This moment is forever etched in my memory—local anaesthetic given, eye taped open so that I don't blink, seeing the scalpel move across my line of vision, and FEELING the surgeon slice my eyeball open. As it turned out, I was resistant to anaesthetic, and the dose given to me wasn't enough to numb my eyeball. They didn't want to insert another needle under my eye, so the only alternative was anaesthetic drops administered directly to my eye and a dose of something through the IV to calm me down—I was freaking out on the operating table! Even after other surgeries, injuries, and giving birth to two children naturally, this is still the single most physically traumatic experience of my life. The surgery on my first eye was done; I would have to come back in two weeks for my other eye to be done. An eye patch was put on, and I was sent home.

The following day, I was driven back to my surgeon, he took off the patch and checked everything out; he was happy with the results, despite the process being less than desirable, and assured me they would increase my anaesthetic dose for the second procedure.

As I left the surgeon's office, it started to rain, and I could see it. For the first time in my life, I could see the rain falling from the sky. Previously, I only knew it was raining because I would get wet and annoyingly end up with water drops on my glasses, but I had never actually seen rain. As my mum drove me home, down a road I had travelled hundreds of times before, everything looked similar but so, so different. I saw leaves on trees for the first time and noticed that they were different shades of green. I noticed the detail in the tree trunks, the variations in the bark. Until that day, they were a blurred brown trunk with a mass of green leaves atop, not dissimilar to how a five-year-old would draw a tree—that had been my reality. I was amazed at the depth of detail and variety of colour in the world, that I had been told about, knew it was there, but just had not been able to see it.

I was apprehensive about going back for the second surgery, but knowing the clarity waiting for me, the intentional disruption was never going to happen. I could finally see! I could see hundreds of meters away; I could see that the hills surrounding my house were not just homogenous blobs but amazing collections of grass, shrubbery, and trees. I never knew so many shades of green even existed! I would tell my friends to run over to a far hill and wave to me, simply because of the joy I experienced because I could see them from such a distance now. Prior to my surgery, if we had been playing in the hills, if they went more than

50 meters away from me, they would just blur into the background, and I would have to wait for them to find me or hope to stumble upon them.

Learning the structure around intuition and how to tune into it whenever I chose, and hear it even when I wasn't intentionally tuning in, was like the cataracts had been removed. What I had been doing, the moves I had been making and the direction I headed had been right, but it had all been blurry, and while I knew there was more out there, it was always just beyond the field of my perception. Not anymore—I finally saw myself and the world for what it was. By embracing my inner voice, I started to gain clarity about my life's direction. The noise of doubt and fear began to fade, replaced by a deep sense of knowing. I realized that intuition wasn't just a special ability for a select few; it was a birthright, an innate guidance system available to everyone.

As I began to trust my intuition more, my life started to change in profound ways. But these changes also came with their own set of challenges. Growing up in a Christian household, I had been taught to place my faith in God and the teachings of the church. My understanding of the divine had always been framed by traditional religious beliefs, and the concept of intuition—listening to an inner voice that might not align with established doctrine—was unsettling at first. I found myself grappling with deep-rooted tensions between my spiritual upbringing and the intuitive guidance I was beginning to embrace.

Exploring intuitive guidance as a way of life meant that I had to examine my beliefs about God and the church. This process wasn't easy. It challenged my understanding of faith and made me question whether following my intuition was in conflict with my relationship with God. For a time, I felt as though I were walking a tightrope between two worlds—the familiar world of religious faith and the emerging world of spiritual intuition. It was a disorienting experience, and I struggled with the fear that I was abandoning the teachings that had once been my foundation.

It was during this period of inner conflict that I discovered the work of Neville Goddard. His teachings resonated with me in a way that few others had. Goddard spoke of the power of imagination, the creative force within us, and the idea that God resides within each of us as our own consciousness. This was a revelation to me. For the first time, I saw a path to reconcile my faith with my intuitive understanding. Goddard's perspective allowed me to view intuition not as a departure from my faith, but as an extension of it—a deeper connection to the divine within me.

Through Goddard's teachings, I began to see that faith and intuition could coexist harmoniously. My intuitive guidance wasn't leading me away from God; it was bringing me closer to the essence of divine truth. This shift in perspective was transformative. I no longer felt torn between two conflicting beliefs. Instead, I realized that following my intuition was a way of living in alignment with the divine will that resided within me. It was a way of expressing my faith in a more personal and profound manner. This reconciliation between my intuition and faith didn't just change my beliefs; it transformed how I practiced my spirituality daily, allowing me to trust in a deeper, more personal connection with the divine.

As I continued to trust my intuition, my life started to change in ways that weren't necessarily visible from the outside—I was still living in the same house, going to the same job, and interacting with the same people—but internally, everything had shifted. There was a newfound sense of peace that permeated my daily life, allowing me to slow down and be truly present in each moment, rather than being consumed by the endless rush of tasks and worries that once dominated my thoughts.

This shift in presence had a ripple effect on my relationships, especially with my children. I found myself engaging with them on a deeper level, truly listening to their stories, their concerns, and their joys. I became more attuned to their needs, both spoken and unspoken, and this led to more meaningful and fulfilling interactions. The once-frequent feelings of overwhelm and frustration began to dissolve, replaced by a calm confidence in my ability to navigate the challenges of parenthood.

It wasn't just about doing things differently; it was about being different. I was more grounded and more connected to my inner self, and this inner alignment naturally began to reflect in every aspect of my life. The everyday moments that once felt mundane were now imbued with a sense of purpose and clarity, and I started to experience a deeper sense of fulfillment in the life I was living. My external world hadn't changed, but my inner world had undergone a complete transformation, and that made all the difference.

As I delved deeper into my inner world, I began to notice a profound shift in how I experienced life. The more I worked on healing my inner wounds and aligning with my true self, the more my external world began to change. It was as if the universe was responding to the transformation happening within me. The relationships that once felt strained started to heal, opportunities that aligned with my values began to present themselves, and the persistent feelings of anxiety and overwhelm started to fade. The old adage, 'as within, so without,' became a living truth in my life. The inner peace and clarity I was cultivating began to reflect in the outer world, creating a ripple effect that touched every aspect of my existence.

It was during this time that I realized it was no longer sustainable to remain in a corporate role that had drained so much of my energy and passion while giving me nothing in return. The time had come to make a change—to step away from what no longer served me and to pursue work that resonated with the person I was becoming.

Leaving the high-stress corporate role that had drained me for years was a deeply liberating experience. The decision wasn't easy, but it was necessary—a step toward reclaiming my life and aligning it with my true self. I had spent too many years conforming to expectations that weren't my own, driven by the need for financial security and the validation that comes from external success. But as I began to trust my intuition, I realized that no amount of money or status could compensate for the toll that job had taken on my soul.

Pursuing work that truly resonated with me was like breathing fresh air after being suffocated for so long. I sought out opportunities that allowed me to express my creativity, connect with others on a meaningful level, and make a positive impact. It wasn't just about finding a new job; it was about creating a life that reflected my values and passions. This shift opened up new avenues for growth and fulfillment that I hadn't even known were possible.

As I made this transition, I also began to address the past traumas that had lingered in the shadows of my life. I recognized that the pain I had endured—whether from toxic relationships, the pressures of single parenting, or the struggles of my childhood—had not only wounded me but had also shaped me into the resilient, empathetic person I had become. Instead of running from these experiences, I chose to face them head-on, embracing the lessons they had taught me and allowing them to guide my healing process. I learned to forgive myself for the mistakes I had made, and in doing so, I found a sense of inner peace that had eluded me for so long.

In the midst of this healing, I discovered an unexpected joy in single parenting. By trusting my intuition, I began to approach parenting not as a burden or a challenge, but as an opportunity to grow alongside my children. I became more attuned to their needs and emotions, making decisions that were guided by love, empathy, and a deep sense of knowing. Our home became a sanctuary—a place of stability, warmth, and unconditional support. I found joy in the small moments: the laughter we shared at the dinner table, the quiet bedtime stories, the spontaneous adventures. These moments were no longer overshadowed by the stress and anxiety that had once dominated my life. Instead, they were filled with the light of connection and presence, creating a loving environment where my children and I could thrive together.

Leaving behind the corporate world and stepping into a life aligned with my true self was more than just a career change—it was a transformation of my entire being. It was a journey of healing, embracing my past, and finding joy and purpose in the present. And through it all, my intuition was the guiding force, leading me toward a life that felt authentically and beautifully my own.

I invite you to start listening to your own intuition. Begin with the small decisions, the subtle nudges, and trust that inner voice. Let it guide you not just toward a specific goal, but toward a way of being—one that is aligned with your true self, filled with peace, clarity, and a deep sense of purpose. Remember, intuition is not about reaching a final destination; it's about living a life that feels authentically and beautifully your own.

I share my story not just to recount my journey but to inspire others to discover the profound connection between intuition and faith. My path has taught me that intuition isn't just a fleeting feeling or a special ability; it's a powerful, guiding force that is accessible to all, a divine gift woven into the very fabric of our being. It doesn't matter where you come from, what you've been through, or what challenges you face—your inner voice is there, a quiet but persistent guide, leading you toward your true purpose.

I encourage you to start listening to your intuition, to see it not as separate from faith but as an integral part of it. Begin with small steps—take time for quiet reflection, pay attention to those gut feelings, and trust that inner nudge. As you do, you'll begin to realize that the clarity and direction you seek have been within you all along, waiting to be discovered. Intuition isn't just a tool for making decisions; it's a way of living, a lifestyle that aligns you with your deepest truths and the divine guidance that resides within you.

Looking back, I see that my life's journey has been about peeling away the layers of doubt, fear, and external expectations to uncover the clarity and purpose that were within me all along. Just as cataract surgery revealed a world of vivid detail and colour, embracing my intuition has unveiled a life of profound clarity and meaning. I now understand that this inner knowing isn't separate from my faith—it is a divine expression of it. This gift, this intertwining of intuition and faith, is something we all have access to. It is the key to living a life of authenticity, fulfillment, and true purpose. Embracing intuition is not just about reaching a destination; it's about living a life that feels aligned, purposeful, and guided every step of the way.

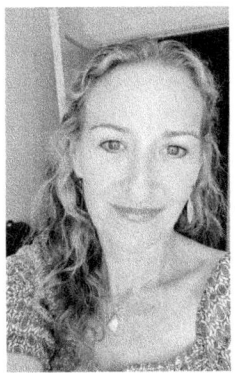

Nicole Farrar

CEO of Wild Hearts Events and Retreats,
Founder Rules Beach Turtle Monitoring

https://www.facebook.com/benicolejfarrar
https://www.instagram.com/nicky_salty_mermaid_adventures
https://wildheartseventsandretreats.co/
https://rulesbeachrest.org/

Nicole is a passionate woman's health advocate. She has been supporting clients to reach their wellness goals for decades in her varied roles. Navigating her own health journey has given her a unique perspective as a patient and practitioner.

Through her retreats, events and mentorship programs the Wild Hearts Village was born. Nicole inspires women to embrace change and transform their health and their lives. She believes that every woman holds magic within her essence that unlocks through connection.

She has a profound connection to the natural world & simple sustainable living, all driven by her commitment to creating a better planet for future generations.

Grounded in her mission for environmental balance, Nicole devotes her time to the preservation of marine sea turtle nesting grounds on the southern great barrier reef where she lives.

Choose Your Own Adventure

By Nicole Farrar

As a child, I loved to read, the choose-your-own-adventure series were my favorite. At the end of each chapter, the reader was given multiple choices: Option A—turn to chapter 6. Option B—turn to chapter 7, etc. The reader was able to navigate the journey as the characters. These books were structured in a way the reader could go back and reread them and choose a different path and the book would take on a whole new storyline. The characters would embark on a whole different journey. Growing up in a country town prior to the invention of the internet, our main source of indoor activities was board games and library books. Looking back, rereading a book and having a different outcome was not only a practical solution to boredom but raised the excitement level considerably. My love of reading is still present, although I'm partial to a great audiobook these days.

* * *

Following my second daughter's birth, I noticed a change in myself. Well, many, really. A natural evolution that comes with motherhood, I'm sure. Although, looking back, the first warning signs were present even though at the time I wasn't aware. I loved being a parent, watching the delight on their faces, the seemingly boundless excitement for the life they had. How they viewed the world from a space of innocence.

To-do lists and ever-growing piles of laundry didn't excite me, a necessary additive to a growing family. On the surface, I rocked it. Although internally, I felt the struggle, the "juggling" that's required as a mother who has many roles. A generally fit and healthy young woman after my last pregnancy (twins!), my vitality didn't return as it had previously. I put it down to having young children under the age of three and shrugged the niggle off.

I joined a local gym to improve my fitness and there I found endorphins, a natural high produced from exercise. Yes, please, I thought, my zest returned, and I was the fittest I'd ever been. I naturally became more sociable: playgroups, twin club, swim lessons and gym classes in between my part-time employment. I took on supporting roles in their dance classes and would take long walks and bike rides in nature. I developed more of a sense of myself and a taste of what had been lacking.

* * *

In 2005, my brother's suicide rocked me to my core. It's never easy to say goodbye to a loved one, we are never ready. The grief took its toll on me, my family and our close-knit community. It was literally one of the most challenging times in my life. The personal torment and years of trying to make sense of it are hard to put into words even now. Grief is a personal journey in itself.

Less than 12 months after my brother's death, I was diagnosed with a serious melanoma. Life turned upside down. I did not have a scenario for this! I was asked to write a will, get my affairs in order and decide who would raise my daughters if the treatment did not go as planned. Sobering and humbling, to say the least.

Aged 32, I was told I had a 15% survival rate, I was scheduled for surgery one week later. In the following months of recovery from the surgery (I was left with around 100 sutures and unable to use my left arm), I was given another shift in perspective. Learning how to take care of my kids and the house whilst regaining my mobility and resting to allow the wound to heal. My mother would drive to my house each morning to make school lunches, walk the children to school and return to shower me and do my housework.

My recovery progressed, as part of the operation was to remove the lymph nodes from my underarm. I diligently did recovery exercises every night until I had good mobility in my arm. I didn't return to the gym as the strength in my left arm took much longer to return. I was offered another position and found great inspiration in teaching over-50s strength training. I would take weekly classes at the retirement village and the local community hub.

Most of my clients were in their 70s and 80s, and wow, they were a great bunch of people. They sure knew what life was all about. They taught me it was all about quality, their goals were to maintain strength, mobility and balance, they loved what they loved, and their goal was to be fit enough to do what they loved. On the surface, things were going well, yet I felt an underlying heaviness present. Like something just didn't quite fit. Months later, my second marriage dissolved, and I told myself it would be easier on my own. The kids and I packed up, moved house and moved forward. This opened up the space to develop a deeper connection with myself.

I began cultivating a spiritual practice. Still at times struggling with the lingering loss of my brother, lack of sleep and anxiety, I looked at my habits and attempted to remedy some of the symptoms I was struggling with. I was finding it increasingly difficult to sleep: my mind would race, and I couldn't seem to unwind in the evening. From the moment I woke tired and feeling like I had not slept. An achy body coupled with a foggy mind and an internal push that had me running incessantly to try and "catch up". I was curious to find ways I could incorporate inviting in more peace. These practices formed the basis for me to slow my mind down, invoke mindfulness and restful sleep. At the time, a single mum with limited resources. I had a job, ran a busy household, took care of four children, and most nights fell into bed exhausted only to toss and turn to no avail. I removed the TV from my bedroom and started lighting a candle or incense each night, remembering to breathe and pause. I started with just a few minutes a day, expanding out to 15 minutes. The monkey mind settled. A whole new world opened for me. I had been concentrating on what I didn't have and what I didn't want.

I had not given so much space to what I DID want. My relief had been sweet and ever so short-lived, a few short months later, I became unwell again.

This time crippling migraines and pain in my body. Barely able to open my eyes due to light sensitivity at times. I struggled to maintain my employment and to be present with the children. The physical pain engulfed me and caused deep emotional imbalances and, at times, crippling anxiety. The cycling health issues took their toll, physically, mentally and emotionally. It felt like one thing after the other. Rolling waves knocked me over every time I found my feet. I had small children that I wanted to see thrive, I wanted a quality life. I wanted to be a model to my children that anything was possible for them. That they could be anything they wanted to be. How could I do that when I was drowning?

I was given medications and returned to work. For a little while, I did all the things, and yet not too much changed externally. I pondered what my next move would be.

My youngest children had just started secondary school. If I could just wait a few years, I could go off on my adventure, and it wouldn't disrupt their schooling. Surely, the health issues would be gone by then. Things improved slightly, enough for me to get serious about why I wanted to adventure. I contemplated why I was putting it off. What was I waiting for? And with that, I called a family meeting (which consisted of everyone at the kitchen table). I shared my thoughts and what I was considering, and I gave them time to think about what they wanted. A few days later, we reconvened at that kitchen table, and they were in! With that, we hatched a plan to move Interstate.

I purchased a map and spent every spare moment organizing what this might look like. Researching where we might go, what roads we would take and how long in driving hours. I created a vision board and decorated it with my wishes for us. Laminated it and hung it on the wall in my bedroom in a place I would see many times a day. Tangibly, it was around 2000 kilometers, I calculated about 3–4 days of driving. Pretty much the furthest I'd ever driven or towed a trailer.

The next three months, we downsized, decluttered and reduced our belongings. We sold everything and kept only what would fit in a small box trailer. We each had a huge case of clothes and 3 boxes of personal items. My eldest daughter had a job and a partner and chose to stay in Victoria. With 3 children in tow, our worldly possessions on board and pretty much no idea how I was going to do this, I set my plan into action. The drive out of town was one of the hardest things I have ever done. With the excitement of garage sales, farewell parties, and trip planning behind me, it all became extremely real. I was shaking and felt nauseous but still somehow holding it together. There was a moment just before we left that I wanted to tell my parents and best friend I had made a huge mistake. I wanted to beg someone to come with me. To scream, I had no idea what I was doing. I pulled the car over ten minutes down the road, crying so hard I couldn't see. I was choking back the tears, but they wouldn't stop. I sent the girls to buy snacks and took a few minutes to gather myself, breathe and give myself a little pep talk. Adventure was what I was looking for, and adventure is what I got. It took huge leaps of faith and lots of deep breathing.

* * *

The GPS sent me over a mountain range on the second day, slightly faster it said, unless you are towing a fully loaded van and trailer. The windy, steep roads slowed us considerably, although the scenery was beautiful. I got incredibly lost on our third day of travel. The accommodation I booked had no trailer parking, which had me park in a grassed area. Torrential rain almost had me bogged down the next morning. Nonetheless, we arrived at our destination a little weary and still very excited to see our new dwelling for the next month.

It looked nothing like the pictures online. It was filthy and tiny, and I could not see us staying for even one night. Absolutely not for one month!

I was exhausted and shocked, sinking to the ground and leaning against the wheel of the car with my head in my hands. What the hell was I going to do, I literally packed up these kids and drove them halfway across the country. Two choices. Stay or go? But go where? Many frantic phone calls later, I found a vacancy for two nights. Asked for a refund and waved goodbye to the tiny, dirty box.

Gypsies it is, then. How romantic, location-free. Reassuring myself it's only for a couple of weeks. It will be fine. I had family a couple of hours drive away, keen to see some familiar faces and an opportunity to store my trailer, which I was still towing, so we set off on a day trip. We drove through a little town at the base of a majestic mountain. It was like nowhere we had seen, straight out of a glossy rainforest brochure, breathtaking and beautiful. As we made our way down the meandering country road, we fell in love. "Wanna move here?" I blurted. There was a resounding "yessss"!

* * *

With the end of the year looming, I needed to get a rental and organize schools and uniforms for the new school year. We spent every day driving to open houses and exploring many areas of the valley. We looked at house after house and drove for hours. I filled out the application after the application. One house stood out for us. At the base of a ridge, it was surrounded by pastures and had a large wrap-around deck with the most magnificent views of the mountain. It was even freshly painted, with a fenced yard and lots of room for that veggie patch I had pictured in my mind. The school bus picked up at the end of the road. Perfect!

There were 15 to 20 applications for each house. I filled in the application, crossed my fingers and waited for the phone call. Just two weeks before Christmas, we received approval and moved into our dream house, sleeping on my uncle's camp mattress as we had NO furniture. We had our new space and I remember staying up really late, the girls and I chatting to each other from our new rooms, filled with excitement and possibilities.

The first-time magic revealed herself to me. After all the mishaps, u-turns and detours, I'd done it! We had our new home and were full of anticipation to see what was in store for us. On the other side of the deep breathing, taking a leap, it unfolded more beautifully than I could have imagined. I used to think the fear would go away with each decision, you know, disperse, the older I got. It never did, and it never does. I taught aerobics for years. I would get the same feeling in my body. Sweaty palms and a racing heart, just like a type of stage fright. The fear doesn't go away, we get better at calling bullshit on it. We settled into our new routine. I secured employment in a retail job, and the girls started at their new school. I would visit my uncle weekly, and on one of my visits, I was introduced to an old friend of his, Penny.

Penny was the first adult I'd ever met who openly spoke about and lived her life by magic. When we met, Penny was in her 60s and an artist, healer, art teacher and guide. In her earlier years, she had been a model and curated a gallery in Tasmania.

Penny lived on the side of a sacred mountain under a huge fig tree surrounded by rainforest in a little double-storey weatherboard home. Her home was filled with antiques and mystical items. Every wall was adorned with artwork, shelves and cabinets filled with crystals, oils, essences and totems from around the world.

Each item was displayed meticulously for viewing pleasure. Penny's love of storytelling was well known by all who knew her. She would light up at every opportunity to share one of her tales. She articulated herself in a way that was enthralling and captivating.

One of my fondest memories of Penny is at her 70th birthday gathering in her tie-dyed dress with her pink-lensed John Lennon-style glasses and a huge smile on her face. We had squeezed all the guests onto her tiny deck lined with chairs and tables overflowing with food. Laughing and sharing stories, her heart was beaming that day.

Upon meeting Penny, a connection sparked, and so began the first of many synchronicities. We would spend hours at her property, making vibrational flower essences and hosting workshops and art classes, it was the most joy I'd felt in a while. My time spent with Penny ignited something in me. I developed a thirst for knowledge. I went on to study energetics and several healing modalities. Knowing and loving Penny, hearing her recall her intrepid tales became my personal inspiration for what was possible. She shared story after story of instances where magic had been demonstrated to her. Of seemingly impossible solutions to problems and miraculous circumstances. Strange synchronicities and how everything just works out in the end.

Penny looked at learning as research. If you do something once and it doesn't work, then you have a formula for what doesn't work. You try again with a different formula, you get a different result. This knowledge we carry becomes a kind of invisible toolbox, you carry with you through the journey of your life. She did her best to live in harmony with the natural world. To work with the earth's elements and natural seasons, cycles and rhythms. To share more love in the world.

A self-proclaimed white witch, Penny would share stories of working in the unseen, with the animals and mineral kingdoms. Of creating with strong intentions for the highest good of all and the harm of none. I can still hear her saying these words as I write now.

* * *

My daughters completed their schooling and moved out, so it was time for me to downsize as I no longer needed my large rental. Time for new views! I found an awesome little spot on the other side of the valley. Decluttering again, packing my belongings, it was a moving day. I was halfway through unpacking the huge food shop in my new space when a car pulled up the driveway. The man got out of his car with a puzzled look on his face. Me assuming he was lost. He asked me who I was. I explained I was Nicky, the new tenant who had just moved in. He paused, looked at me and exclaimed, "I'm the owner of the house and I didn't approve a new tenant. My son is moving in." Shocked and a little confused, we conversed. The old tenant had sublet to me without the landlord's knowledge. I spent the next two days relocating, storing my belongings with friends.

I found a space temporarily, a caravan with a tiny deck and annex. It was cute and comfortable. It became my temporary home for the next two months, not exactly what I had gone for. At the time, I was horrified and could not make sense of the circumstances. Some blessings don't look like blessings straight away. The journey of the days that unfolded from that caravan was synchronistic. I landed in a cottage amongst the rainforests. A run-down frame house at the base of the Great Dividing Range built entirely of hardwood timber. We named it, "The Little House on the Prairie." My partner at the time and I set to work clearing and repairing the house. Planting vegetables and flowers. Creating a home amongst the rainforests.

It was paradise. I would often laugh to myself at the crazy circumstances that found me in my dreamy location. Recollecting all of the times it looked like it was all going downhill fast. If the other rental had worked out, I would never have found my little house on the Prairie. My paradise.

I had always secretly wanted to live near water. This property had three creeks bordering it, and a quaint driveway entrance over a little wooden bridge. My favorite of the creeks ran across the back of the property, completely secluded from everything. A short stroll a couple of hundred meters from the house was the entrance, like stepping into an enchanted forest. Huge hundred-year-old hoop pines bordered the creek, and native ferns and gingers bordered the rock walls covered in moss and bracken.

The crystal-clear water from a natural spring was icy cold. There was a series of rock pools peppered through the creek, rearranged with every flood. I spent hours watching the water weave around the rocks and settle into small pools. The sound of the water was mesmerizing with dragonflies and butterflies circling above the surface of the water. Coming to rest on the rocks. It became my happy place.

* * *

Physically, health challenges resurfaced. Physical pain returned: migraines, muscle fatigue, brain fog and rashes that did not heal for months. Itchy, burning and weeping wounds that needed constant care. I rarely left the house as the changes in temperature and wearing clothes would aggravate the sores. I visited the creek twice a day and paddled my feet in the cool cleansing water. Patting the water on the rashes, attempting to soothe the constant itch and sting. I would sit in the middle of the creek, cry and pray for relief. Drifting to sleep at night sobbing, I would wake up the same. Basic tasks became a challenge. Showering myself and cooking were exhausting. Many doctors, tests and seven specialists later, I received my diagnosis.

Fibromyalgia. Dubbed the invisible illness because it affects and presents differently in each person. Having had years of experience with clients and now having done years of my own research, the best description I've come up with. It affects the fascia in our body. (Which covers every muscle in our body.) It predominantly affects the nervous system in some patients. I was told there was nothing that could be done for me. My GP would keep an eye on things. I was advised to manage my symptoms as best I could and take pain medication when I could not manage. I was 46 years old.

Which now, looking back, was the catalyst for yet more change.

* * *

After the shock wore off, and oh so many reflective conversations with myself, I figured I was faced with a choice again. I could give in to my diagnosis and yield to my current health reality. Wither away and, eventually, die quietly. I would require care and services to look after me as I wasn't coping well on my own. Or I could put what energy I did have into rewriting my story and creating a different outcome. Become my own medicine and Guru!

* * *

"The secret of change is to focus all of your energy not on fighting the old, but on building the new." Socrates. I read the note on my fridge for the longest time. My mantra and a reminder.

The little house on the prairie was sold a short time later; my time in that paradise was gone. It was time to move on. Amidst a pandemic, I said goodbye to my sanctuary in paradise, finding myself with no destination. Navigating border closures and storing belongings, I was back in the car with a trailer. I traveled, staying with family and friends and framing the whole thing as a prolonged holiday. No definitive plan. Following my heart, which was extremely fragile at times, much like my body at the time, the stress took its toll.

I trusted that I would land exactly where I was meant to. Honestly, it wasn't full trust every day; it was a pendulum constantly fluid between "I got this" and "What the hell am I going to do?" It gave me an opportunity to reconnect, manage my health conditions in a different way and, most of all, relearn how to take amazing care of myself.

I house-sat, helped with my grandchildren, volunteered where I could and focused deeply on what I dubbed radical self-care. Radical self-care differs from what we generally consider taking care of oneself. It encompasses the tough decisions required to move quickly through where you are and where you desire to be. Seeing my own patterns and where they don't serve. Needing to rest regularly, I dived into online programs and got curious about the root causes of disease and the underlying connection with our stored trauma and body. How our experiences shape the body. The mind-body connection and how to rewire it. I worked with mentors to support my health goals, and what I wanted to create moving forward.

* * *

My days became about rediscovery and getting to know myself on the other side of the transition. Mother, wife, partner and all the roles that were so familiar to me had fallen away. I was solo for the first time since I was 18. Joining circles and workshops and engaging in creative arts, connecting deeper to my intuition and cultivating habits from a space of joy. I reflected daily. If I really did get to write this next chapter, if my life was a blank canvas, it had to be a masterpiece.

What would I paint?

What did I love, and where did I want this to go? The "traveling" went on for almost three years, this time was full of new experiences. Sunrises in new locations and lots of time spent looking at the stars. At times, feeling like they were my only constant. Resistance, pain and lots of things that didn't feel like they were working (on the surface). Full surrender to my inner compass as my guide. Being okay with questions that I didn't always have answers to. Framing it as an adventure contributed greatly in those times when I felt directionless and lost. It's only in hindsight that I'm able to see these experiences were my formula for growth and the pathway out of the loops. For me, it was time to skip chapter 6 and choose my own adventure!

* * *

Armed with my invisible toolbox of wisdom gathered from my years and my desire for change. But how, with a "broken" body, no stable home base and the logical odds looking like they were not on my side? I had to follow my heart.

Focused on what I'd love to create, I got really clear on what and where. I played with what it may look like. I missed living immersed in nature, running with the natural rhythms of the seasons. A simple and slow more intentional lifestyle that would support my well-being and quality of life long term. The first time I'd watched a sunrise over the ocean was in a coastal village called Rules Beach. Listening to the sounds of waves and tides. Huge tree-lined skies filled with stars, happy place vibes to me. I had been visiting this area for the last few years and falling in love. Not long after my first visit, I came across a turtle carcass that had washed up at the entrance of the beach. I had never seen a turtle that big in real life. Too heavy for me to move, feeling great despair that this magnificent creature was dead, and no one was around to notice.

My friend found a lovely local man, and he removed it with his tractor; he said it was common that they washed up. That same day, whilst strolling along the water's edge, the idea came to me: Maybe I could help the turtles? The sea turtles nested on the beach around the point. They had been returning for decades each nesting season to their place of birth to lay their eggs. Most programs were run by volunteers, and Rules Beach did not have anyone actively monitoring. I dreamed of living with the land, helping the turtles, and recreating my slow simple life.

* * *

Focused on the action that would support the turtle program and myself long term. So much more than a turtle program, this space would be a community space, my personal home base and headquarters for turtle monitoring, a village! And it pretty much took off from there.

In 2023, I purchased acreage minutes from the nesting grounds. The block is in various stages of regeneration and is a new adventure of learning for me to explore. I opened a section as a campground, and it's lovely to share paradise with travelers, family and friends. We have big plans to expand and build. The rich birdlife, the roar of the ocean at high tide and the campfire glows really stand out to all who visit.

It's our second year of data collection. We work with nearby community-led citizen science groups in conjunction with the Queensland Great Barrier Reef Conservation Association. We are little fish, but when we all do our bit, we create ripples of change. It has been a huge first season and year of growth, both personally and for the turtle project.

I aim to host online circles, experiences, workshops and gatherings, supporting women in doing what I have; well, their version of it. To navigate the mysteries of wellness and to create a life beyond their wildest dreams.

* * *

Embodiment practices help me to keep the balance of being and doing. If someone had told me a decade ago that I was going to find my medicine in the fresh air, dancing and gentle stretches, I would have laughed my head off. For now, my fibromyalgia is manageable most days. I am living independently and learning to thrive.

Wisdom often comes with experience, and decades of poor health, doctors, tests, certificates and modalities have shaped me into the woman I am today. Doing the inner work, meeting my own creative spark, my inner muse and how she fits into my adventurous story has made a profound difference.

She is a version of myself that feels vulnerable to show to the world. A true dreamer with rose-coloured glasses who wants to paint the world with love. At times, a sassy, salty mermaid who daydreams about living in an enchanted underwater garden. For now, she is happiest in her little cottage by the sea.

When I find myself in a space that I didn't expect, I will often use my humor to shift focus. Yelling, "Plot twist! Grab some popcorn!" Treating life with lightness and curiosity continues to serve me. Like this is a blockbuster movie, and we've just hit the bit where the story shifts and takes another turn. The story takes on a new direction, and the plot thickens.

Looking back, I see the magic and how it unfolded FOR me to form my story. When things were seemingly falling apart, there were greater things at play.

There is great wisdom in the dark gifts of our life. When judgment, grief and shock fall away, we are left with acceptance and a new lens to view the world. All this forms a rich tapestry that becomes the masterpiece that is our life, our unique story.

* * *

There is a way out of the cycle of chronic illness, but you won't find it in a diet, pill, fad or healthcare professional. It is not one-size-fits-all. It will be unique to you, your body, your life and your circumstances. The pathway is an inward journey, one of radical exploration of self and full expression. Of undoing, unlearning and shedding. An honoring of the past, the presence and a healthy curiosity for the future.

Would I write my story the same way again?

I don't know. We are all dealt the cards of our lives, and like all good card games, how we play them is our choice and determines the outcome. Some you win, some you lose. In the end, it's the polarity of our experiences that makes for a colorful story. It's sometimes through the hardest of times our true spirit shines through. My story was always meant to be big and bold and filled to the brim with all the things. Like any well-written plot.

I just had to have the courage to live it.

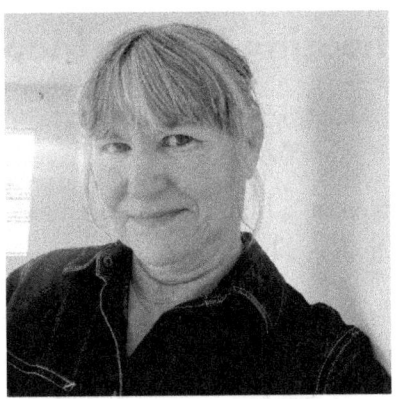

Caroline de Burca

Coach, Homeopath

https://www.facebook.com/caroline.deburca
https://www.instagram.com/carolinedeburca/
https://www.muckandmagic.com/

Caroline, a Homeopath by day, an Anthropologist by training and lucid dreamer by night delves into the mysteries of the mind and the nature of personal reality. Her passion for Homeopathy and Anthropology has led her on merry dance to both inner and outer space as she unravels the intricate connections between the physical and metaphysical. As a lucid dreamer Caroline navigates the boundless landscapes of the subconscious to unearth her deepest truths and sees the extraordinary in the everyday life.

As an anthropologist, she has immersed herself in cultures around the world, unearthing the sacred rituals and ancient wisdom that connect us all. Whether deciphering the mysteries of the subconscious through lucid dreaming or delving into the healing properties of Homeopathic remedies, Caroline is driven

by a boundless curiosity and a sincere wish to understand, navigate and master the human journey.

Shooting for the Moon

By Caroline de Burca

I had a friend who lived on a boat on the canal in London. I said to her one day, 'I'd love to live on a boat.'

I was finishing my degree, preparing for exams, and writing a thesis. Wrecked, tired, and I was broke. And the lease on our house was up. And as it happened, my friend rang me and said there's a boat here if I'd like to take it. There was a 55-foot-long narrowboat called Madam. I lived in it pretty much rent-free for three years. It was a charmed existence. Mobile phones were not a thing at the time, except for the London City financial boys. It was the size of a brick and weighed as much. The battery lasted 4 hours. On the flip side, it was too big to slide out of your back pocket and down the loo.

I used to paddle the canoe across the canal to get to the tube station. It was a 5-minute walk over a bridge. But we canal dwellers often used it for the fun of it. I fell in one morning on my way to work and had to go back to shower and change. So, I was late. My boss said that was the best excuse he had heard in a while.

I decided I wanted to live in a house. On the surface of things, that looked impossible given my means. But there was an energy there of determination, a soft energy. I knew I was going to do this. I engaged the services of a financial advisor and set about finding a property. I bulldozed through a lot of obstacles, some of them gracefully. I employed a financial advisor called Neil Armstrong. I called him the Moon Man, as I really was shooting for the moon. To cut what could be a long story short, I bought an apartment, number 13. I knew when I went to view it that it was mine. It was perfect for me. It cost 55,000.

When I was asking about which mortgage I should choose, Moon Man said it doesn't matter. 'You'll only be paying your mortgage for a couple of years and then you're going to win the lottery.' It was delivered as a statement of fact. You could have blown me down with a feather.

That idea took hold of me. And it was working like a worm through my energy field, throwing up all my judgements and notions about how life works.

I had always wanted a life with horses. And if they could somehow fund their large appetites—hoof care, vet bills, and general well-being costs—all the better. They are big pets, in some ways as expensive as children, except that you can't leave children out in a field at night.

Those who seemed to be in the know about such things, i.e., owning horses, said if you want to be a millionaire with horses, start with 2 million.

An acquaintance of mine organized an event to introduce Amma the Hugging Saint to Ireland. She asked me to help with the hosting. Hugging Saint has a huge energy field, and you can get really clear really fast in her presence. As I was waiting by the stage to receive my hug, which is how she gives her blessings, I was asked by one of her minders if I wanted my question answered in English or Irish. I had no idea I even had a question, but I realized I did. 'What am I doing on the planet?'

I had my hug and was about to leave the stage when one of her orange-robed swamis tapped me on the shoulder and said, 'Amma said you are to sit on the stage and meditate.' Which I did because I am a good girl. Some awareness washed over me and said, 'Create heaven on earth and go straight there.' That seemed sensible enough. And with that, the same swami tapped me on the shoulder and said, 'You can go now.'

And just in case I hadn't gotten the message, a lady handed me her business card, which said, 'Co-creating heaven on earth.'

I was walking on the beach one day with a friend. It was too windy and cold to swim. And I said I'd love to rent a movie and have baked blueberry cheesecake. I changed my trajectory slightly, and with that, I kicked a stone. What looked like seaweed was actually a €50 note. You can have what you love at the speed of light.

I had a very vivid, lucid dream one night. I was watching a young girl who I had known as being on the spectrum, so to speak. Not sure if that is the correct nomenclature these days. Anyway, she was riding around in an arena on a horse backwards with her eyes closed. That struck me as odd because it is odd. The dream felt very significant.

Later, I received an invitation to a Zoom call from an acquaintance about a little-known equine therapy. Intrigued because of my dream, I hopped on and learned about something called Alpha Brain Balancing, which involved rebalancing the brain by riding around in a circle on a horse backwards with your eyes closed.

I was glad to know that my dream was not a metaphor for how I was living my life. I would have generally agreed that it felt like I was blindly going round and round in circles, and backwards to boot.

So now I had a mission, something to aim for.

Lockdown came, and I was working as a nurse. I knew I needed to stay happy and healthy so as not to be infected by the fear and insanity going on. And as I was an essential worker, I was free to come and go. I bought a campervan. It was a vintage Hymer. I called it Dinky. It had everything you could need to live comfortably and a lot of funky little things: flyscreens, blinds, a little bathroom, a kitchen, and a bed over the cab. I always felt like I was on holiday when I drove it, even when I was going to work. It had a big steering wheel, and I was always happy bopping along in it.

I got busy with all that was involved in setting up a business with horses. And when the time came to buy horses, I sold Dinky to my neighbor who loved it as much as I did. He said, 'I love it, it's so dinky.' He had not known that that was its name. It had gone to a good home.

I bought horses. Well, I bought Dilly as my therapy horse, and Buddy came with her as a companion.

I knew that I had bitten off more than I could chew. I was very aware of it and I was on a steep learning curve. But having fun sometimes.

If you want to break a man, buy him a horse.

I missed Dinky. I had a hunch to enter a competition to win one. Tickets were cheap, a tenner or so. I bought one. Draw day came two weeks later. I came home from work, and I thought of it. I looked for my ticket number. I wrote it on a piece of paper and left it on my bedside table. I believe I spoke it out loud and asked it to come to me. I went to bed and fell asleep. The phone woke me at 11:30, and I knew before I answered it that I had won. And indeed, I had.

I couldn't get back to sleep, so I phoned my sister and told her about my win. She told me to take the money as I hadn't had the time for both the camper van and the horses. I knew she was right, so I took the money and hoped the universe wasn't auditing me.

When I was looking for my ticket number, I remember saying I'd love it. And there was an energy there, a very warm, open feeling, peaceful, expansive. A fullness, a delight without attachment. I can't replicate it necessarily spontaneously, but the energy was definitely inspired by the love I had for Dinky.

Now I had some money to invest in my alpha brain balancing business.

Nothing happens by chance, or so says the Kybalion. I asked for it to come to me and somehow I had rearranged my molecules so that it showed up. In the two-week period between buying the ticket and the draw taking place, the idea of the campervan was working its way through my energy field, looking for all my objections and judgements of why this was just not possible. I attended to all these thoughts and judgements and gave them their proper place and put them to bed.

Doctor Dean Radin of the Institute of Noetic Sciences has been looking at the relationship between mind and matter, specifically, intention and attention and its outcomes. And as it happens, reality shows up biased towards your attention and intention.

There is a book written by a PhD called *The Art of Luck*. In it, he describes the characteristics of lucky people. They're optimists, they listen to their intuition, they leap at opportunities, and they are resilient. I would credit myself with those qualities.

I have done a lot of wandering in my life. And not all who wander are lost. But I have certainly gotten caught up in the doldrums or an eddy or circling the drain hole. There's a difference between fixing oneself and course correction. Go straight there to your heart's desire. Connect the dots. Sometimes it might seem that there's a long time with a lot going on, but nothing happening. Keep straightening yourself out by making choices. It's all magic, or none of it is, so says Einstein.

I stopped to ask for directions from an old man. Walking down the road. He looked like he had weathered many storms. He said in response to my query, 'Well, now I wouldn't start from here.' He was just shooting the breeze and killing time. He had his arm in my window and he was not going anywhere in a hurry. And it now looks like neither was I. His hilarious response had me pondering. Where was I generally coming from? Wrongness. I'm wrong, you're wrong. It's all wrong. You get the picture. Any road will do if you don't know where you're going. I knew vaguely what I was heading for. Start where you are. There's no other way to do it. I generally wanted to be anywhere but where I was.

I have an inbuilt homing pigeon. My brother lost his phone on his two-acre lawn and it was turned off. But I knew exactly where to go because my body knew it's connected to everything through all time and space.

The first time I went to a cranial sacral therapist. As she touched my head, I felt like my strings had been cut. I didn't necessarily know what that meant. It was a feeling. I felt like a sack of potatoes with no clear direction. What became clear with time was that all these strings were my conditioning. Life is like a pattern that keeps unraveling to the point where all judgement concepts, good and evil, disappear. Then you were left with the fabric of the universe. Knowing has a sense of peace and space. And you can flow with that. Surrender. And things can take shape. Follow your dreams, nourish them like they were your baby. Follow through on your gut feelings and intuitions. You can have what you love.

I have noticed that I usually have a big energy shift before something pays off. I was driving in Asheville, NC. To me, it was the wrong side of the road with the steering wheel on the wrong side of the car. I had to really reorient myself in time and space with a new spatial awareness. And had to do it on a second-by-second basis. I had an address but not the help of Google. And as I was being spaghetti hooped around Asheville lost, I decided to ask some parking angels and hoped I wasn't pulling them off jobs. I followed my intuition and I got to the right place. It turned out it was their new home. With no signage. And it was not the address I was aiming for. But somehow, following my intuition, I got there. Easily.

To get through life with intuition, it will get you there and it can be easy.

On a trip to Costa Rica, I attended an impromptu workshop on the Flower of Life, which invites you to connect with the universal patterns of existence. The Flower of Life is an ancient symbol found in many cultures, and some say that it is the fundamental blueprint of all life. It consists of a flower-like pattern of overlapping spirals. And as we drew ourselves in and out from our core, every time gaining a new awareness. Maybe the Hokey Cokey is what it is all about.

Of course, the doubt, dithering, and delay never left me. Never leaves me. It was a constant companion. I asked myself one morning as I was going to work, 'Can I really do this? Can I really win the lottery?' I kicked something on the ground. It was a coke can. It was one of those that had a limited run. There were names on it like you, me, us, them, and maybe others. I picked it up and it said you, it was a 'you can'. I was like, OK, the universe has answered me with a you can. That made me laugh. The universe has a sense of humor. It shows up when you are aligned with what's possible for you. The world works as your oracle. Make up your mind. Turn yourself around and bring yourself to it.

Apparently, I'm very impressionable. And sometimes, I put that to good use.

Lovely spacious meditation with a friend one evening. And as I was leaving, she gave me a bag of damiana tea, which looked like a bag of grass. She said jokingly, as I was leaving, 'Don't get pulled over by the police and spend the night in a cell while they test the tea.'

On my way home, I stopped at some lights. It was a quiet night. And then I did what I never do. Picked up my phone. Didn't engage the handbrake. And started scrolling. Then I heard two car doors slam in front of me. I hadn't even seen the car. It was a police car. And I had rolled into it and hadn't even noticed. Two police officers walked towards me. What part of my consciousness played that little trick on me? Dropped an idea into my head and somehow I created it. Now could I put a good idea into my head?

Every so often I needed to get comfortable in my own skin. And not take my issues so personally. They act as a cookie cutter for you to carve you out of infinite space. That's where you start, and the rest is up to you and your choices. There is an energy to the ask. If you look at the energy when you're asking, you can hear it. You can really hear yourself and know where you're coming from.

Are you Star Trekking where everybody's been before? And there's no room. Or are you connecting to your true space, which is internal? Spelunking.

I asked someone once who was well-versed in the art of metaphysics, 'If you know something is possible, how do you make it real?' She said, 'You have to ooze into it.'

Addictions had an agenda that kept me distracted. I was defining myself by the emotional range of my childhood. Most of me was stuck back there. You get an awareness to integrate, you move on until there's enough of you here and now, in the physical reality, in some sort of coherent shape to receive what you're asking for. Order has intelligence.

Your awareness and your knowing bring you there. Stop distracting yourself and create space. That contributes to your knowledge. It's an energy shift. Focus on what you love, not your problems or your issues. It takes practice, like going to the beach and cold dipping. It used to take me a long time to get in. Now in a couple of breaths, I dive in. Sometimes it takes practice. Or you could just do it. Nike was right. Knowing has a sense of peace and space and boundless flow with that.

It takes a lot of energy, power. To leave the gravitational grip of the collective and your own past. But if you can lighten your load, you can move at warp speed. So the more stripped of baggage you are, the less rigidity you create, the faster things can move. The intensity needed to reach a goal is there once you decide. Get out of the sluggishness of your normal functioning.

We had an elderly family friend who was quite sweet but could be painfully pedantic. She asked me to do her shopping one day as she was not feeling well. With a list as long as my arm and even longer instructions on how exactly she wanted her vegetables to look. I set off muttering to myself, 'She is driving me up the wall,' and I did, in fact, end up on a wall, from a dead stop at a petrol pump, firmly perched on a low wall that was parallel to the car, with four wheels spinning. It looked impossible. Four guys from the nearby car wash picked it up and set it down. Those guys still give me a wide berth when I meet them.

So what sorcery mustered the forces?

When shooting for the moon or the impossible, you need to readjust every second because everything is in motion.

I sat down on my meditation cushion one day, with the intention of creating heaven on earth, and was wondering what that would look like. I was very serious.

I was practicing a meditation I had learned from the work of Carlos Castaneda. I have studied anthropology and was fascinated by his books. In this meditation, you are guided to find a point on your back and enter into your heart and rest there, then ask your heart what it wants. My description is lame, but the meditation was wondrous.

I asked what it wanted and was immediately informed that it wanted to win the lottery. I laughed out loud.

I had a lot of notions about what I should be doing. I was a product of my upbringing and felt like a mass of unchecked spawn growing in every direction, glop and glup, that sticky stuff that will keep you bound to the past .

 It was the idea that would not go away and I was treating it like a big problem and certainly not as a possibility.

I was at a place again where I needed to up my game with this whole horse thing!

I asked the universe for a hand. I bought some rubber gloves; there were three in the pack, one orange, two yellow, and all different sizes. They leapt out at me because they were so tightly packed. Someone on the production line got distracted. It happens.

Cleaning is what I do when I don't know what I'm doing. My life might be a mess, but my house is clean.

Ooze into it.

Can I be brave enough to claim the future I would love? Or continue to regurgitate the past and be distracted by bright shiny things? Be present and deal with what's in front of you skillfully and turn your attention to your dreams.

The current reality is just data. In a week where I was particularly discombobulated, I met two guys within a couple of days, both called Cosmos. What are the odds? I needed to tune in.

Come home to myself and quit blundering around Wonderland, I knew enough.

Life is like a pattern that keeps unraveling to the point where all you thought you knew for sure is just not true. Mark Twain said it better.

Stop being nebulous with the universe. What happens in vagueness stays in vagueness. The message needs to be clear and free of conflict—load your arrow with your knowing. And sculpt your path out of the void in your own inimitable style. Energy needs a direction. It needs a job.

Look at the energy of the ask, it has all the information you need to course correct. And then you realize you are awed by the peace and space, and you sometimes can't stand it.

On one of my days when I felt like a wanderer, I borrowed a book from the library and went to the beach. I planned to swim, but I could not put the book down. It was *The Life of Pi* by Yann Martel. It is the story of a boy, a tiger, and a shipwreck. Pi was being interviewed by insurance agents when he finally made land. They did not believe that he had spent years on the high seas with a tiger in a small boat. As Pi pointed out, no one believes they can win the lottery but someone always does. And as he then says, so it is with Gods, they like a good story.

I went to the fairground with my nephew and niece, and surprised myself by going on the 'freak out' ride instead of the joyride. My choices weren't great.

I needed my molecules rearranged, I used a product from Aura-Soma called the Humpty Dumpty bottle, which realigns your energy field and it certainly did. I was in the bathroom after putting it on. It's a very pleasant oil, and I was not expecting what happened next, I felt like there was a tornado raging around me. I heard banging and glass smashing, it was very dramatic. I could feel my molecules weaving back and forth and finally settling in the center.

There is a song by The Verve which was my anthem for a while: 'A hundred different people all in one day, it's very confusing.' Bits and pieces of me all over the place all with their own trajectories and stories. Conscious coherent energy exerts a stronger pull and magnetizes things to you. It really is a matter of lightening up and getting yourself together. Choices muster the forces.

Pi is a perfectly repeating pattern, life is a spiral, you can go up or go down.

One thing I've noticed is that spirit (because I have a degree and a firm grasp of the obvious sometimes) communicates with me through my eyes. If something catches my eye, I know I need to pay attention. Sight is active, not passive. I have found a place for me and my horses and my business.

I know what I'm aiming for. I'm pulling the trigger on that one.

Where is the money coming from? Wherever it is now.

So with the knowledge of how you are put together comes the responsibility of this newfound freedom and space. I am wandering around my consciousness and staying present with my choices and bringing myself to them.

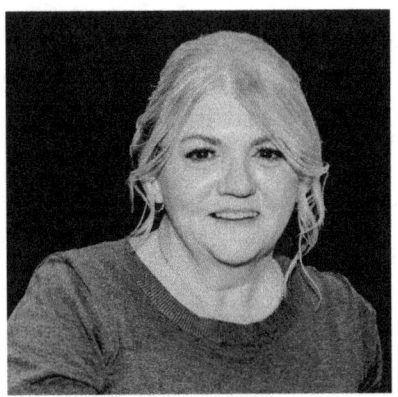

Jo Cathie

Founder of MMC Coaching
Coach

https://www.linkedin.com/in/jo-cathie-88181a15/
https://www.facebook.com/profile.php?id=100089762430095
https://www.instagram.com/mmccoaching
https://mmccoaching.com/

Jo Cathie embodies the principle "know thyself," specializing in mind-body-soul healing through subconscious exploration and re-attunement to oneness. With over 25 years as a holistic healer, energy worker, and intuitive guide, plus 15 years as a professional chef, Jo offers a comprehensive approach to wellness. Jo has spent years studying the relationship between food frequency and its ability to raise consciousness, enabling access to higher bodily intelligence and unleashing intuitive guidance.

Jo's proprietary process leverages her gifts as an energy channel, medium, and body healer, effectively aligning mind, body, and soul while releasing fear and restoring oneness. Her transformative workshops, meditation classes, and innovative Dancetation energy movement sessions have positively impacted numerous lives.

In "As If By Magic," Jo shares her personal journey, illuminating intuition's power in facilitating rapid, positive change. Jo offers readers a roadmap to self-discovery and personal empowerment that creates lasting change through Jo's experiences and insights.

The Awakening -
An elevation of Consciousness

By Jo Cathie

I write this as a dedication to my oldest sister, who passed away in January 2024 of metastasising brain tumours. Fiona Anne, I love you, and I thank you for the incredible gift you gave me in your passing. Sisters forever.

As I sit to write this chapter, a feeling of incredible joy, peace and happiness permeates my heart and spreads a delicious warmth throughout my body. I can actually feel the earnestness my partner John is experiencing from the other room, he is perched at our kitchen bench, searching the internet for the perfect holiday park for our Xmas getaway.

I am aware of Holly, my dog, snoring lazily on the veranda. She is happy and content and exudes that energy whilst she sleeps. I hear the joy of the birds outside my window singing their song. Most importantly, I am aware of and can feel my connection to the oneness that flows to and through my heart and connects me with every living creature on this planet.

God, the universe, your higher self, your superconscious, call it whatever you will, but know that it has such a funny way of putting you on track when you are out of sync. At the time, it can seem like everything is coming at you at once, and it is the worst experience of your life, when in reality, it is the unanswered prayer you have been desperately searching for.

I don't even recognise myself now, it happened so quickly and as if by magic. It was like I flicked a switch and was reborn, keeping the wisdom of the past without the pain and the trauma that had plagued me from childhood. Sometimes I pinch myself to make sure I am real, it's the most amazing feeling. Stepping into this new version of myself, happy, joyful, vibrantly alive, living as a true expression of my heart. Creating a life that I do not want to miss a minute of.

I can assure you, it wasn't always this way.

Becoming Numb

I was 4 years old when a family friend of my mother's came to stay and the sexual abuse started, my innocence was stripped from me; my childhood stolen.

It stopped around age 13 when I started my period. I believe he was afraid I might become pregnant, and he would be caught out. I look back now and realise that is when the numbness started, it was not when the abuse stopped, though, I continued to perpetrate that on myself for the next 40 or so years.

Growing up, my stepfather used to call me Wonder Woman, and would often say to me, "How do you fit everything in, you've got so much on your plate." What he didn't know is that I loaded my plate so full in an effort to drown everything out, for it was in the stillness that the past would haunt me. That gripping fear in the pit of my stomach, the voices of shame, guilt, embarrassment, doubt and insecurity that ate away at me, stealing any joy until eventually they ruled my entire thinking.

I felt trapped in a life I couldn't escape from. I had tried therapy and done the whole merry-go-round of the Western world in order to find some peace. I had tried forgiveness and every spiritual practice out there, and yet, still the voices in my head persisted, the numbness invaded my soul. On the inside, I was craving for a future that deep inside I knew was possible, for a level of joy and happiness I desperately longed for, a deeper connection to myself and others.

I was overrun by feelings of worthlessness and never enough that had pervaded my soul to the point that the only way I could stop it from eating me alive was by keeping myself numbed out. I did alcohol, cigarettes, and at times, abusive relationships, trading one form of abuse for another, all to feed the inner demon that continually told me that I was useless, worthless, and damaged. No matter what, I couldn't shake the belief that there was something innately wrong with me, I was faulty and that is why I had been abused, with thoughts of 'I didn't deserve to live' or 'I shouldn't be here' constantly running through my mind.

Add to this, I was born with the gift of mediumship, and the ability to have what is almost an X-ray view into people's bodies and energy fields, in short, "Bodies talk to me", which is something that I didn't really understand or integrate until a few years ago. Using this gift as a 5-year-old child and not knowing what was appropriate to say or not, with no filter, got me in loads of trouble and only further perpetuated the belief that there was something wrong with me. I don't belong, I don't fit in, I just couldn't figure out how to get it right here on this planet.

By age 7, I had created a vast network of subconscious programming that was running the show, and I didn't even know it. On top of that, there were the thoughts in my conscious awareness that I did know about yet didn't know how to change, like old familiar friends they played on a tape loop: "You're not good enough", "There is something wrong with you", "You don't belong here", "You're a misfit" and "You will never amount to anything."

For my entire life, I have been on a never-ending quest to "fix myself" and find peace in my thinking, as I truly believed at my core that I must be faulty and broken.

Fast forward to 2018, my partner John and I made a choice to invest money into a new business. We did so under the influence of alcohol and the coercion of a family member, never a good time to make any choice. Long story short, we followed bad advice from an accountant, and the family relationship soured; eventually, the company was liquidated, and we lost everything.

All of John's superannuation we had withdrawn to start the business was gone plus everything we had in savings. At the time in our lives when we should have been thinking about semi-retiring, we were dead broke, feeling more defeated and broken than ever and believing there was no way we could ever recoup the money, buy a house or repay the debts.

John fell into the depths of depression, and at times, I was afraid he would take his own life—things got so dark. I just kept working, I was in shock, I didn't see this coming, and a level of disbelief and numbness crept in that was even deeper than anything I had ever experienced before. Underneath the numbness was that old familiar sense of shame, guilt and embarrassment. In truth, I wanted the world to open up and swallow me, I just wanted to disappear.

I had to keep going, I had no choice, I felt like a machine on automatic pilot. Rinse-wash-repeat, every day felt like Groundhog Day with no end in sight and no brightness of the future.

I kept thinking surely there is more to life than this, there must be another way. I craved to find it, to feel alive, engaged and connected. I couldn't—I drank copious amounts of alcohol in the hope that I could forget how much of a failure I felt like, to forget that I had given up on my dreams and, more importantly, so I couldn't feel how much my heart truly hurt.

It was around this time that, quite by accident, I stumbled across an amazing book on structure and magic. Even the way it showed up in my life was truly magical, and it did so at a time when I was probably at one of the lowest points I had ever known.

Having spent years working in natural therapies previously, I was using all the tools I had in my playbook to shift my headset around what had happened with the business breakdown, nothing was working. I couldn't pivot out of this one, and I was also trying to support John, who was drinking and smoking heavily and had stopped communicating, he was in shock and numbing out. Eventually, I admitted to myself that, like John, I too wasn't coping, I was depressed and was on the verge of giving up.

John took a job back in WA, and we had to temporarily relocate. To make the long drive shorter, we listened to e-books to pass the time. It was during this trip that we found ourselves listening to *The Secrets of Natural Success*. I loved the concepts and premises in it so much that I decided to study more about structural tension and the art of creation. This led to revealing a core egoic belief I had that I was prey or actually worse than prey, I was shark bait. The end result of this belief was that I was hiding from life because I believed the world was a cruel and horrible place, which to that point had pretty much been my experience even though my genius nature, my soul, the truth of who I am at my core, wanted to be fully expressed in life.

Learning about this underlying belief and the structure I had been living from started a chain of events that changed the course of my life. I engaged in the tools and applied the work, I learnt a lot, changed a lot and started to create my life in a whole new way. Money was flowing in again, I was feeling much happier, we had repaid most of the debts and John and I were in a place where we could see that it was possible for us to buy a house. John had shifted out of depression, had also created a high-paying job with a great roster and had some spark back.

I was also using the principles and tools of creation and intention in my workplace as a holiday park manager. Over the course of the next 3 years, I made significant increases to the revenue month in and month out. My boss gave me a raise and a bonus and still to this day asks me, "How do you do it, Jo?" At one point, I had to provide an explanation for the significant increase, which made me laugh with pride at my achievements.

I was now working with a coach, as I felt encouraged by my achievements and wanted to take them further. I was hosting creation events in her group, growing in confidence, being of service and starting to shine. I was bringing my own unique brand of magic to the world and the women I worked with were feeling the difference. Life was good, and a level of happiness was creeping in. I felt good.

In January 2024, I received the call that my oldest sister had passed.

At first, I didn't feel anything when I heard the news. I just said, 'Thank you for letting me know', and hung up the phone, no sadness, no grief. I didn't really feel anything at all, we had been estranged for a few years, and I was angry at her for wasting her second chance at a new beginning. I had saved her life many years earlier when I had found her in a prescription painkiller-induced unconscious state, she was bent over on all fours trying to start the fire and had passed out in a position that had cut off her airway, and she had stopped breathing.

I couldn't feel grief or sadness, but I could access anger. I stomped around for several days in this state until one evening, a few days after leaving this earthly plane, Fiona came to me in a dream, gifting me with an understanding of the pain that had filled her life, her despair, her emptiness, numbness and disconnection and the fear that had held her captive since she was born. She showed me others like her and motioned for me to wake them up. I didn't understand this, and I recall asking in my dream, "How am I going to wake them up, I feel the same way."

I woke up with a strange sense of relief but quickly forgot about the dream. I did, however, make a clear decision that no matter what it took, I would not waste one more second of my life being controlled by the past.

Fiona had lived a half-life, joyless, suffering, never truly living and that broke my heart to see.

In that moment, I committed to a life of no regrets, I committed to myself, I committed to knowing absolutely everything there is to know about myself, my subconscious mind and how to create the fully engaged, lit-up-joyful-over-the-top fun life that I had been craving, that I deserved, that I was born to live. I committed to sharing that with the world and teaching others how to have the same.

I had made huge steps forward; however, this experience, the numbness that had crept back in with the news of her passing, had shown me there was still something missing.

I'm a naturally curious person, I have always believed in the saying "know thyself", so I became curious about why my sister died and why I didn't, why I couldn't feel anything. Cognitively I did, physically there was nothing. I had been in such judgement of myself about this, yet soon realised this was not a one-off experience, that same numbness had happened repeatedly in many areas of my life, including when my father passed away when I was 18 years old, when my horse died and then again in 2019 when we lost the business.

Something told me this was deeper than just a structure, it was a total annihilation of my beingness from a state of body trauma so deep that the only coping mechanism I had was numbness. My gift has always been bodies, so now it was time to gift to mine. I had already noticed a pattern/structure every time I stepped out in the world to shine my light and do my work out there in the world, my body would be wiped out with illness. It was time to put on my detective's hat and find out what was going on.

I had a deep innate sense that whatever it was, it was the core of everything, and unravelling it would set me free.

Now, I realise that sounds all very pleasant, but trust me, it didn't actually unfold that way, I was about to release a three-month program called 21 Ways to Love Your Body in the weeks prior to Fiona's death. I was excited, it was like birthing a baby. This work had helped so many women have breakthroughs with their bodies, and I was teaching them how to communicate with their bodies and create new relationships with their bodies using structural tension, energetic principles, superconscious recode techniques, subconscious reprogramming and my own unique magic called Dancetation. I believed in it. I was excited.

True to the unconscious structure I had been experiencing around stepping out and being seen, I broke my ankle in two places and totally immobilised myself a few days prior to the launch. Like seriously, now I was beyond curious, this pattern was so obvious that I had to find out what it was that was keeping it in place.

Shortly after Fiona's passing, I was talking with John about it. I threw my hands up in the air in a gesture of surrender and yelled out, "WTF! Universe, angels, whoever is listening, I give up! For years, you have been trying to get me to work with these gifts, and now I am finally ready to do so, and this keeps happening, what more do you want from me?" Ok, I will be honest, it was a bit of a rant; however, I needed to express it.

I was now acutely aware that even though I had changed my financial area using the tools I had learnt from my mentor and my coach, there was a deeper layer that I had until now either refused or been unable to access owing to childhood trauma. Something I had buried so deeply it was secret and hidden from me.

I also realised that since the crash in 2019, I had rebuilt my life: I'd get up, go to work, run circles or meditation classes, smile and laugh, and I would now have fleeting moments of connection, but I couldn't actually maintain it.

For all intents and purposes, my life looked really good from the outside: happy relationship, high-paying job, beautiful family, gorgeous grandchildren and good friends. To everyone who knew me, my life was successful again, as if 2019 hadn't happened.

But it wasn't.

At my core, there was still something missing. I still felt disconnected, like I had been unplugged from life and as desperately as I tried, I didn't know to plug back in, only now I was tormented by the fact that I was experiencing the fleeting moments of the lit up, engaged, connected and joyful life and I wanted that as my full-time way of living.

Working with the principles of structure had taught me that I wasn't broken, that we set up structures, or belief systems if you like, and these run in the background governing our experiences. Some are core foundational beliefs that orient us here on planet Earth, others are learnt beliefs we have adopted during our childhood from experiences, incidents or our parents, teachers and the like. Some of these beliefs served us when we were young, but as adults, they are outdated, outmoded and of no value.

I have always believed that our thoughts create our reality and had spent a lot of my life working diligently to change mine, lord knows I needed to with what I had been through, and now I was learning to take that a step further. When I integrated the learning that your Focus Creates your reality, I realised that the problem is that what most people think they are focused on is not what they truly think they are focused on. Most of us are focused on getting away from pain, not moving towards pleasure and end up attracting into our lives more of the very things we are trying to avoid.

I realised that the majority of my thoughts were about "not having" things I didn't want instead of being about how to bring about the things I did.

For example, in the past, I had an underlying belief system that I was prey, shark bait, and the world was a cruel and horrible place. I formed this belief system as a defenceless 4-year-old child being preyed upon by a sexual predator. In that moment, my cries for help went unheard, and no one came to my aid—hence why I believed "You can't rely on others" and "The world is a cruel and horrible place."

Without awareness of this structure, my focus was on avoiding more of the same, which inevitably created more of the same. Repeat experiences of people I couldn't rely on showing up, being taken advantage of and not seeing it coming.

The clarity this gave me in regard to the experiences of my life was incredible, but it didn't release the numbness or disconnection I was feeling.

It wasn't until my rant at the universe and my surrender that it became clear.

I am often woken at all hours of the early morning with the inspiration to do something or listen to something. But on this particular morning, all I did was reach for my phone and suddenly it started playing all of its own. It was 4 am, and I didn't want to wake John, so I quickly put on my headphones and shoved the screen under the blankets so as not to shine the light. A thought popped in, "You've turned your light out." I was like, wait, what???

Then, I closed my eyes and continued to listen to this woman talk about releasing fear. She rattled off a couple of questions that you could use to stimulate your journaling that would help with writing it out and some other useful tips. I fell asleep and forgot about it for a few days.

During that time, I saw the word FEAR everywhere, it was like my superconscious, Angels Divine guidance, whatever you want to call it was telling me I needed to look at fear.

So, I did a ramble on what I knew about fear and all the obvious things, for example, fear is the absence of faith, we aren't born with fear, fear just limits us and holds us back. I need to learn to be aware of and manage my fears. Fear is a signal that we can use as a signpost, it isn't real. Fear is activated by the amygdala, if I learn to use it properly, I can turn fear into fuel. Then, I wrote out all the things I knew I was afraid of, and that's when I got it.

It isn't what we know about or what we know we are afraid of that stops us; it is what we are unaware of, all of the things that we hide from ourselves, that we keep secret hidden and invisible. So, how do I access the truth of FEAR? I asked out loud and then I remembered the Cathartic Writing Questions. I combined them with a process I learnt years ago called the meaning process and the end result was incredible.

I woke early the next morning and started writing it out.

It blew me away, and my life has changed forever.

The first sentence I wrote was:

"Fear means never having any fun." Well, that was true—my life had not really been fun since I was a child. In fact, I didn't even know how to have fun, despite craving it.

And then it went on from there...

Fear means creating ways to fail,

Fear means feeling disconnected,

Fear means feeling powerless,

Fear means feeling like a victim,

Being no one,

Never asking for what I want,

Fear means missing out on life,

Fear means wastage, wasted time, wasted life, wasted energy,

Fear means a broken heart and an unhappy life... Yep, got me, I had been living that one!!!

I wrote until I had nothing left, and then I wrote some more. I could barely keep up with the pen. The words just flowed, and by the time I had completed the series of questions, I realised I had written easily and effortlessly for almost two hours.

In the closing few sentences, I wrote—"I don't have fear in my life as it is no longer necessary."

Because it isn't real,

Because I am no longer choosing it,

Because I know I am divinely guided and protected.

I don't have fear in my life. I have peace, love, gratitude, ease, joy and fun.

I don't have fear in my life because I am whole and complete; I am oneness. Source energy flows through and to me.

When I sat back and read the words on the page, I realised that fear was a program that becomes activated when our brain (mind) has a perceived threat of something now or in the future that could be life-threatening.

The brain (mind) or egoic structure has one job in life: to keep us safe and keep the body alive. Let's face it, you can't play on the earth without a body.

The mind is the conscious part of you, the thinking brain, your soul is your genius connection to the universal energy or oneness that we are all connected to, and both, the mind (ego) and the soul (genius), occupy a body in order to play on the earthly plane.

In his book, **_You Are the Placebo: Making Your Mind Matter_**, Dr **Joe Dispenza states**, "_Just as thoughts are the language of the brain, feelings are the language of the body. And how you think and how you feel create a state of being. A state of being is when your mind and body are working together. So your present state of being is your genuine mind-body connection._"

So, it makes sense then that if the mind has had its fear circuits activated by either a real or perceived threat from pre-birth to age 7, the trauma response kicks in, and it will shift into survival mode and do whatever it can to keep the body safe, including the body's ability to feel. The numbness, unplugged, tuned out, half-life disconnected feeling becomes the norm, and some people never know any different.

Far too often, we ignore or abuse the body, which also blocks the ability to feel, instead of recognising the incredible magic the body has to offer and listening to its intelligence.

The soul's connection to the mind is through the body, the soul-heart connection point is inside the body behind the physical heart and about one inch down. When the mind shuts down the body's ability to truly feel, it automatically cuts off the connection to the soul and, in essence, dims our light or connection to oneness.

The Bible speaks of the mind, body and soul. I have spent a lot of my life on a quest for the integration of mind, body and soul, and suddenly in front of me was a road map showing me how to integrate all three and wake people up to their oneness. Suddenly, I recalled what my sister showed me in my dream, and I understood what she was showing me and what the thought, "You've turned your light out", actually meant.

No one does this to us, we do it to ourselves, mic-drop moment.

I quickly wrote a short workshop to take this out there into the world. I was so excited I wanted to share it with everyone. The first workshop went off without a hitch, then the second, then the third, and so it goes. No more being wiped out by my mind disabling my body. I had freed myself.

I had seen the moment I had dimmed my light, and I had turned it back up. Re-attuning and waking up to oneness was like coming home, the incredible joy that flooded my entire body was indescribable, and every day since has been one of joy bubbles, immense gratitude and happiness.

I can feel things on a deeper level than ever before and I love it. I actually feel lit up, like a phoenix rising from the ashes, the pain of the past has transformed into wisdom and the numbness has disappeared. The clarity of my heart and its desires and what it truly wants to create is crystal clear and I can hear it's calling.

Following it, being guided by it, living with the synchronicities that wondrously show up and lead me to the desired end result can truly only be described as Magic.

It is like sunshine and air, it is free, it is available, and all you have to do is believe in magic.

It has been almost eight months since that dream moment. Every day since has been filled with joyfulness and a greater sense of happiness and zest for life than I have ever experienced. I feel a deeper sense of connection with myself, my body and my life, and that deep inner craving for change has been realised.

I'm not saying every day is perfect, I still have to interact with people who are acting out their own programs and trauma patterns. What I can say is how I deal with these is what has truly changed. I don't make them mean anything about me, I'm not triggered into fear and the automatic responses and programming that used to rule my life. Instead, I am easily able to observe and witness without judgement of myself or others. I can respond to situations from my heart instead *of* reacting to them. The other major change is that the nagging voices in my head no longer haunt me on a constant basis. I can look in the mirror, and I know that I have fallen in love with the woman who looks back at me. I know she is strong, intelligent, worthy, capable and amazing; I really like her.

I could say that I have only recently founded this transformational process, yet in hindsight, it has been my life's journey, and the unfolding of it over the past months into a system that can be used to help others transform their lives has been an incredible journey in itself.

I give thanks and unending gratitude to an amazingly magical woman and dear friend Sandra Kearney who has joined me at MMC Coaching. Together we have been riding the wave of conscious magic, following our guidance and intuition to reach deeper heights of understanding around the trauma response that dims us from our light and how to reignite your heart and turn your light up. This body of work chose us, and we are honoured to be bringing it to the world.

Is it time you flicked the switch and turned your light on?

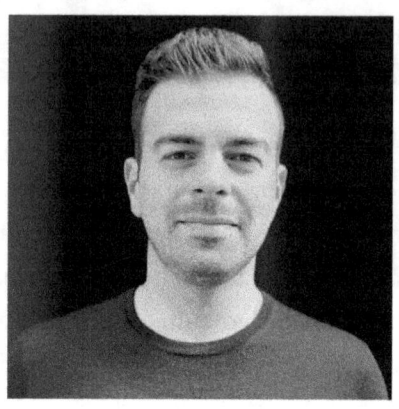

Jordan D'Urbano

Coach & Facilitator

https://www.linkedin.com/in/jordan-d-urbano
https://www.facebook.com/jordan.durbano
https://www.instagram.com/jordandurbano
https://linktr.ee/jordandurbano

Opening myself to living my via intuition has proved to not only be one of the greatest decisions I've ever made. But it has helped me connect to who I really am at my core and let go of who I am not. Coming from a chest beating sales and business environment, where everything was about money and accolades. I've found myself embracing my new life as an author, song writer and coach. If I'm not writing a chapter for my next book, or a chorus for my next song, you'll usually find me running events and retreats for my coaching & education business. Here I specialize in teaching people how to orchestrate a life that they truly love through leveraging creative structures & principles.

Mistrust

By Jordan D'Urbano

PART I:

From the rugged streets of Bali to the cool rainy alleyways of New York City, right through to the rich architecture of Rome. For much of 2021, travel was a beautiful allure that opened up so many doors to information that you just wouldn't have known existed. Places that were dark and depressing, as well as places that were enlightening and incredibly innocent. Depending on what your intention is, travel can shine a light on it all. It can help you acquire such a deep level of self-knowledge that a "new you" can emerge within a very short space of time. A you that is filled with fresh dreams and desires that are beyond what you ever thought possible for yourself.

So when your identity as the "slick and charming salesman" is challenged by the emergence of a dream to create emotive hip-hop music and an online coaching business based on elevating consciousness. Travel not only becomes a time of self-inquiry but a time to create what doesn't yet exist.

At first, you treat everything you create as an experiment just to see what happens. Shortly after, you become curious about what would happen if you began sharing your work more publically. And before you know it, you look up to see that your dreams are beginning to manifest in real life. Your songs are being listened to by a few hundred people a month on Spotify, requests for your free coaching offer continue to pour in. All while you continue to hop around the globe in complete disbelief at how quickly things are changing for you. Of course, you're not making enough money from music or coaching to be absolutely certain that you've made the right choice. Yet there's a curiosity about where this could all go.

However, as the demand for both music and coaching gradually increased. There was an almighty amount of resistance to taking the necessary action to further its growth.

So, rather than focusing on building paid coaching programs or sending songs over to DJs and producers of radio stations, unnecessary amounts of meditation, planning and journaling filled the calendar.

You think you're doing the right thing because you're neutralizing your insecurities around putting yourself out there. But what you fail to see in the moment is that you are quickly becoming addicted to staying safe in perpetual preparation rather than taking direct action to make your dreams a reality.

Here's a snapshot of how most days began to play out during the extended sabbatical.

Dawn would start with an incredible morning routine that would consist of visualizations, strength workouts, cold showers and music to fire up the engine. A few posts would then go on social media to spread the good vibes in the hope that your followers give you an extra kick of momentum with their support. As the high would then tingle your bones and muscles, you're hopeful for a powerful day, where poetic songs are written, your dream coaching offer is created, and if you're really fortunate, you end up bumping into a Mediterranean princess while sipping your espresso at a cafe around 3pm. Yet, hope and intention are two very different things, and as the clock begins to approach 12pm, you begin to see that the pendulum of emotions and thoughts begin to swing back viciously in the other direction. You experience yourself going from high and almighty directly into a melting pot of doubt, fatigue and fear.

When you're travelling, there's an easy cure for this: get out and be a tourist. See everything, eat everything, meet everyone and convince yourself, "Ahhh, that's better. Just needed a break." As long as you're feeling good, there's no problem, everything will take care of itself.

But the reality is, it doesn't. And by the end of what felt like a dazed and disorientating 2021, travel had gone from being medicine to an incredibly unhealthy addiction.

What had at first cracked open the door to a hip-hop career that birthed two albums and a small fanbase, what had helped kickstart the early stages of a new coaching business. Had now become a tool to run away from creating this new life based on real passion and purpose.

You work so hard to create new ideas, new pathways, new opportunities, and though, at times, you don't expect any of them to fly, eventually, they do when you stick with them. So when the day that you've been waiting for finally arrives, there's enough evidence and momentum to suggest that it's time to ramp up your commitment to your music and coaching. If it's no longer making you feel blissful or inspired, and it's not paying you very well. You begin to question whether you made a huge mistake in leaving your well-paying sales job behind.

It's here that the toxic cycle continues, as you look for another dose of "bliss & calm" to lift you out of the doubt that is swallowing you whole. Rather than seeing that you are on track and making progress, you assume that you are failing because your wildly unrealistic expectations of success are not being met.

When you are that blinded, you look for help. You try therapy, you try meditation, you try all kinds of "personal development" based things to compensate for the low sense of self-esteem that you are feeling. But when you spend all your life savings on that stuff, and you look to see that all you've created are short-lived projects and serious doubts about your sense of direction in your life.

You are ready for action. You've created so much tension and energy that you'll either seek to resolve it by leaving this world.

Or by creating something you truly love.

Thankfully, when you have wise people around you, there's always an opportunity to wake up and create a new reality. A reality that is consistent with your purpose, that sees you taking action towards a vision that doesn't require you to be "bliss & calm" all the time. In fact, you can be experiencing both "light and dark" emotions, yet, you aren't fazed because you are focused on something bigger than yourself.

One of those wise people was William Whitecloud, the author of *The Magician's Way*, *The Last Shaman* and *The Secrets Of Natural Success*. His books and courses on using intuitive awareness to create a completely new reality come through in the clutch moment. It didn't feel great listening to what he had to say, yet, it was undeniable that his teachings were exactly what needed to be heard and embraced. One of the things you learn early on in his courses is how to use intuition to tune into what is "true" for you when it comes to making a decision.

Amongst all the darkness at the time, one of the main sticking points was not knowing where home was. When you've gone to stunning countries like Spain, France, Italy, England, Indonesia and the USA, and there isn't one place that you feel like calling home for a while, there's only one solution. Keep travelling.

Yet, when you're out of money and completely fed up with listening to the intoxicating hit of "bliss & calm" emotions to guide you, you are prepared to rely on the more subtle nature of your intuition.

So whilst sitting in a villa in Canggu, Bali, an intuitive exercise from one of William's courses was undertaken all to receive an answer on whether "it was true to continue travelling."

Within seconds, a "no" came through.

Another premise William teaches is that when you apply intuition to make big decisions, your ego is going to come in and resist, almost immediately. So even though you feel horrible about the answer and the fact that your "blissful" hiatus has now ended.

You hold your ground.

What was even more disheartening during this first experience using this intuitive work was the answer that came in for the next question.

"Which location is it true to live in next?"

Like clockwork, you relax, centre yourself and go through the same exercise.

And yet again, within seconds, an answer came in, without any explanation or justification whatsoever.

"Melbourne."

The one place that many Australians were very dissatisfied with at the time. Yet, when you're directed by your intuition, you never question it, even if you feel incredibly resistant towards its answer. You go with it, all while holding the assumption that it's got your best interests at heart.

PART II:

Surprisingly despite all the resistance and apprehension in coming back, landing in Melbourne proved to be a very calming and grounding experience. It had become obvious from the moment the plane touched down, that somewhere deep inside, there had been a yearning to come back. To the familiar surroundings of where you grew up as a child, where you innocently experienced all your firsts.

Kicking your first football, catching your first bus to school, kissing your first girlfriend or even just laughing hysterically with a group of mates prior to a long night out on the town.

It's memories like these that reconnect to your child-like innocence. And though this freeing orientation begins to help you ascend above all the crap going on in your life, very quickly, a voice comes in to kick you down for thinking you could be that person once ever again.

"You are out of money, how do you think this woo-woo state is going to help build a profitable business??

"You are at least 20 kg overweight, it's time to lock in and get serious!"

Of course, everyone's voice is different depending on their current reality and past experience, but this is just a snapshot of how taunting the ego can be when you begin following your intuition. Yet, though the ego's voice got louder, a willingness built up inside to reconnect to the child-like spirit lying dormant within. In William Whitecloud's courses, you learn that the gateway to the intuitive orientation is innocence, where you have emptied out your thoughts and feelings, and are literally imagining that you are looking at the world for the first time.

It's an orientation like no other, though it's calming, there's a subtle anticipation to it. You're not only freeing yourself from the clutches of your ego, but you are also opening yourself up to the subtle intuitive messages that are available to you at all times. The interesting thing about innocence is that it is quite easy to access. It does not take hours of meditation, copious amounts of breath work or an extensive journey on ayahuasca. Though there's nothing wrong with these practices, they are not necessary when it comes to cultivating innocence.

At first, you play around by testing innocence out in a familiar setting, like the forest just near your family home. Though you've been there thousands of times, experienced its beauty through all seasons and seen the same regulars over and over taking their daily walk. When you cultivate innocence, different aspects and themes on any given day jump at you. After being so addicted to experiencing new cities and languages literally every week, innocence was a game changer in seeing that the ability to "start fresh" was always available.

After you experience it in the forest, you then begin to implement it with things that may be a bit more challenging. Like the new green and lush diet that was to be followed. In essence, the foods that were consumed in this diet were actually really tasty. But when you've been so used to the pizza and pasta from Italy, or the delightful buttery and crispy bite of a croissant in France, salads, chicken breast, salmon, and soups come across as very ordinary.

Nevertheless, when you eat these foods in innocence, you begin to notice what you love about the meals and, more importantly, how much better your body is feeling. Rather than being in mourning for all the carby and fatty treats that you are now missing out on, you are in tune with the delight of feeling healthy and vibrant. And, of course, it wasn't long before all the weight began to fall off.

You hear it often: If you're struggling with life in general and things aren't going your way, start with your physical health, and the rest will follow. This proved to be true to some degree, as a creative flow for a new chapter in music opened up, and a fresh circle of friends was established. However, there was still an almighty amount of resistance towards truly committing to building an online coaching business.

Every time you'd sit down to do something for it, a crippling amount of doubt and fear would come in. For at least two months, you'd sit at your desk in the study where you built your first business at the age of 18. You remember all the pressure and angst that you felt back then to be successful, even though you are now more experienced and resilient. The old demons that you swore you'd slayed when you became a success in sales re-emerge hungrier than ever to beat you into submission. As the page titled "Potential Client List" stares at you, the obvious task of writing names of people who fit your market begs for your attention. You write all but five people down before deleting them because you believe, "Why the hell would they want to buy this junk?" You call on innocence to help you follow through, and though you hold it for a few minutes, it isn't long before your ego crushes it, like a kid stamping on an ant.

Even though you know it's true for you to build this business. Overcoming resistance to move forward was proving to be incredibly difficult. And so, rather than taking action, most days were filled with working out, playing the piano and hanging out in the forest near Mum's place. Without knowing it, the orientation of "preparing to act" had surged back, only in a different form.

And so as the inaction begins to undo all the momentum you initially built, you slowly find yourself being involved in other people's problems. It innocently starts off with getting a little interested in celebrity drama on social media. Then you move on to chatting to friends about their problems and what you think they should do about it. And before you know it, within the space of a few short months, you have found yourself busy caretaking for a list of people. What is crazy about this, is you actually get convinced that you are creating magic, because all of a sudden you are needed! Business has actually gained momentum from out of nowhere, lunches with women from dating apps have filled up the calendar and binge-watching sports with mates has become a regular thing.

Of course, there are always symptoms and feedback that are there telling you that you're off track when you're stuck in this cycle. Like when you're awakened in the early hours of the morning to a whisper from your intuition, telling you.

"I want you to slow down and reconnect to the true attributes of the relationship you really desire..."

Or when you do an intuitive exercise to tune in to whether it's true for you to sign a particular client. You get a "no", but proceed to go for the new business anyway.

Though it's subtle, it is clear enough for you to recognise that you're off track and that you're taking the easy way out. At first, it's fine, as you use the excuse you've only been back in Melbourne for four months, you need money and dating is a numbers game. But before you know it, four months is six months, and then six months is a year.

And so a business was built, a fictional book was written, some new songs were stored away on the Google drive and a few flings had come and gone. Decent creations, but nothing that really suggested that life was in flow and on purpose. However, an intuitive thread to go to Central America had emerged. And with the financial pressure slightly easing off in the background, and a "yes" coming through in an intuitive exercise to fly out to Mexico City. The Central American trip was booked for the January of 2023.

Though you don't know why you're going, you assume that it's because there's some magic for you to create over there. Potentially in the form of more clients, the dream relationship, the hit song or even a new destination that felt like home. And though you get excited about the possibility of creating these things, what you don't notice is the desperation behind it. You don't recognise that behind all of those familiar "bliss, calm & hopeful" emotions is a huge amount of impatience desperate to force these things into being.

What was crazy was that everything that had been envisioned, from the house to the location to live, the girlfriend and the clients, all manifested on this trip in the form that matched the vision!

However, as you're trained when you're first learning about intuition, it is highly recommended that before you involve yourself in anything new—a new business deal, a new relationship, a new lease on an apartment, etc.—you are encouraged to tune in to whether it is "true" for you or not.

Regardless of how certain you are, that this is "THE" opportunity you have been waiting for or rather that this is a REALLY "bad" idea. You tune in, always.

So when a beautiful connection came out of nowhere with a girl in our tour group in Costa Rica, it was obvious that an intuitive tune-in was required. Though the ego was absolutely convinced this was the opportunity to create the dream relationship and make real sense of the trip to Central America, you surrendered, dropped into innocence and asked the question, "Is it true to explore a relationship with this woman?"

To much frustration and disappointment, in a matter of seconds, a "no" came forth.

You know you're meant to follow through and assume that this answer is what will best serve not only yourself but the other person, too. However, when you need to make sense of why you feel so strongly about someone and why you have created yet another "fling".

You judge your intuition as wrong.

And so you tune in again, unconsciously sabotaging the whole process to get a "yes".

Luckily, the lust and holiday romance wore off quickly enough, so no moves were made across the world, as it would have more than likely created unnecessary drama.

On the back end of the trip, while hiking through the mountains of Guatemala, an intuitive thread came up in a visualization to move to Lake Atitlan. For those of you who don't know, Lake Atitlan is a stunning body of water in a massive volcanic crater in Guatemala's southern highlands. Beautiful cities on the mountainsides surround the lake giving you uninterrupted views of the water the majority of the time. To no surprise, the second the search for longer-term accommodation began, a house high up on the mountainside of Lake Atitlan showed up. It was literally the first house on the Airbnb listings. It fit the price bracket desired, the views of the lake from the kitchen and living room were stunning, the furniture inside looked incredible, and it was available to rent for three months.

With only a few days left at the current accommodation, it made sense that this might indeed be the opportunity to create a new home. Though there was an incredible amount of resistance to moving to a place like Guatemala, the judgements were parked, and the intuitive tune-in went down.

Though the nerves and anticipation were high, the practice of connecting to the state of "innocence" freed the mind. And the question, "Is it true to book this apartment for 3 months?" was brought into the imaginary circle.

A "yes" came through.

You would think the lesson had been learnt.

Instead of booking the beautiful apartment, a flight to a random Mexican city called Bacalar was booked. Upon arriving there within the short space of two days, a terrible virus was caught. Delirium, diarrhea, vomiting, aches. Everything you could possibly think of, all hit the body.

When you get this sick, and you know what you know about intuition and conscious creation, you want to slap yourself for going against your truth, because you see that this would never have occurred had you just followed the guidance that had dropped in.

Part III:

Jogging down the beaten path is a journey that can seem like it's going to require more courage, confidence and self-belief than usual. You hear of people taking these alternative routes to make their dreams a reality. You're enthralled by their story, yet in many ways, shocked at the amount of supposed "risk" they took on. You hear about the trials and tests that came their way and how they valiantly passed them. And by the time they share how their result came to life, you may have bought into the idea that they have something you don't. And that the only reason "magic" actually occurred in their life was because of their relentless "blissful & calm" attitude.

Upon returning to Melbourne, with a very sensitive stomach and an incredibly sleep-deprived mind, it was tempting to buy into this very story.

When you begin following your intuition, it's easy to think that if you do not follow through on the guidance you get in that VERY moment, the ticket to uplevel in a major way will be lost forever. It sounds crazy, but in this instance, this was the ego's story.

Not only did this add a lot of pressure to be perfect. But it created a crippling sense of scarcity around what was possible. And when you're carrying that kind of energy around with you, even if you do follow through on the intuitive guidance you get, it's likely you'll completely sabotage it.

So post-Central America, though you know that "follow through" is the key to unlocking everything you could possibly want, there was still a major misunderstanding around following intuitive guidance. Though the guidance would come in, heavy expectations and pressure for it to produce results quickly plagued the pathway forward. When you're struggling to apply a modality like this, quite often, you try to make it more complicated than it actually is. After all, it's easier to add or change things, rather than just going back to the basics.

Receiving and following through on intuition guidance is actually quite simple. Have a vision, acknowledge your current reality and allow the tension/space between the two, to compel guidance forth. Follow through on the guidance without any expectations and allow your vision to unfold in front of you.

This is what you're taught, and though, you've had fleeting moments where you've witnessed the magic of this structure. If it doesn't completely change your life or eradicate your problems overnight, you begin to overcomplicate things. So over the coming months, the calendar filled up yet again with extras to help with follow-through. Cold showers first thing in the morning, breathwork, yoga, extra intuitive practices, more time in the forest, playing music and chanting out loud.

You don't know it at the time, but you're once again in the cycle of "perpetual preparing" rather than just following through. Soon enough, the majority of the year had blown by once again, and not much at all had been created. In fact, not only had the creations completely stagnated, but life in general was actually getting worse. You start to notice that your friends, family and coaches are getting frustrated with you. You feel the waistline of your pants tighten, you notice your bank account balance is quickly heading for zero, clients begin cancelling their coaching agreements with you, and you wake up to unexplainable aches and pains in the body in the middle of the night.

Your same old washed-up ideas to grow your business, write your songs and start your second book continue to drop in. You take action on them because you believe it's your intuition, and though they fall short, they miraculously come to visit you again.

You get to a point where you think your intuition has got it in for you. Like it's playing some sick and twisted game to stop you from moving forward in your life. And though you hear the familiar ghosts of the past growing in strength again, the assumption that keeps you in the game is: "Attempting to fix your problems only makes them stronger. If you want your reality to change, focus on taking direct action to create what you love, rather than to fix your problems."

And so problem-solving was dropped. The inessential activities based on "preparing" or "planning" were cleared out. And though it was scary at first to face an overwhelming sense of the unknown, there was this assumption that things were about to change in a major way. You aren't sure how, but with the heightened sense of anticipation and clear intention to only take direct action, you begin to see things that you wouldn't usually see. And after a few weeks of being disciplined for not doing much at all, a golden opportunity landed out of nowhere.

A friend from Canada had just come to visit Melbourne and had shared that she was house-sitting while on her travels. She mentioned how much she loved it as it was helping her save money on accommodation and allowing her to work on her own business in quiet spaces. It turned out that she was using a particular website to find and apply for these house and pet-sitting gigs, which were really popular in Australia.

For whatever reason, house and pet sitting stood out as an opportunity. So, if you think there's some action you should take to help you create what you love, you tune in intuitively, get your truth and follow through on whatever it is.

The lesson had finally been learnt. That night after seeing her for lunch, the tune-in happened and a "yes" came through. The very next day, a few applications had been sent to house-sitting listings that stood out. And in no more than a week, two house-sitting gigs were secured. A small win, yet a very important one. It was a reference as to how quickly something can be created when it's true for you. From here, more pieces of intuitive action steps dropped in, such as taking singing lessons, drinking celery juice, singing in front of a live audience, going to a house sit out in Australian farmlands, solo wine tasting and finally, the most random of them all, heading to Gosford in New South Wales to live for a few months.

Each of these threads was not pleasing AT ALL to the rational mind. And though the ego continued to cry about money and boredom towards living in Australia, you will yourself to park your concerns about your problems to the side and focus on moving forward no matter what.

While consistent income streams and a long-term home hadn't been figured out just yet, there was an evident change. The violent mood swings had stopped, the ego's attempts to cloud follow-through had lost their power, and there was this quiet assumption that everything that needed to be known, would be known in the moment.

A game-changing intuitive thread that once again made absolutely no sense at all was to start painting. When you go through school hating the thought of painting, doubting your terribly fine motor skills and thinking that the practice itself is only good for messing up your clothes, there is a HUGE amount of resistance to pick up a brush and remain open to what the activity may gift you.

Nevertheless, on a Friday night in early January of 2024, a "paint and sip" was booked. Before arriving, a strong intention to create an image of a magical landscape was set, using the initial intuitive guidance as a reference point. Though you don't know how it'll turn out exactly, the focus was placed on the feelings that would arise as a result of the painting. Again intuition was used to get the "true emotions" that would be felt once the painting was finished.

So, though you get the intimidating stare from the blank canvas, daring you to start and not screw up, you remember that initial intention and the feelings that accompanied it. Before you know it, the colours are selected, and the brush starts to move. The whole way you think the picture is going to look like a five-year-old painted it. But you implement what you've been taught by consistently acknowledging what you're focused on in your current reality and willing yourself back to your vision. All while holding the assumption that because this action step came intuitively, there's hidden magic at play.

And after about two hours of engaging in the internal battle of focusing on your vision rather than screwing up, all while continuing to move your brush. You see a canvas full of flowers, with a river stream and a background of green lush trees. You take a step back, observe the picture and almost instantly, the feelings that you set out to feel, arise. It is here you know you've created something from out of nothing.

Leaving the workshop that night, thousands of parallels were drawn between painting and business, painting and attracting the dream relationship, painting and songwriting and even painting and travel.

To say painting alone was what changed everything wouldn't be completely accurate, but to say that it provided a key reference point for following intuition, would be. A few months after, while in Gosford absolutely loving my new short-term home, an intuitive thread to head to Spain came in. Business had really started to take off, a second book was gaining serious momentum, and debts were quickly being paid off. Taking off to Spain at that time made absolutely no sense, in fact, it very much seemed like it would completely crush all the momentum and magic that had been built. However, with all the reference points that had been accumulated, booking the one-way ticket to Barcelona was a complete no-brainer. All the lessons from the past trips had been learnt and it was clear the time had come to experience travel in a completely new orientation.

And as this chapter is being written to you, from the sunny city of Cadiz, in the South of Spain, two months of the most magical trip around Europe has unfolded. From seemingly out of nowhere, not only has the majority of Spain been travelled, but places like London, Amsterdam, Munich, Cologne and Milan have all been visited. Portugal, Greece and France are next. As for the creative momentum, it hasn't stopped at all, if anything, it's gone to a whole other level.

You never know what will make the biggest difference in your life; you never know what simple action step could set you up on a path of magic.

But if you're open and willing to listen to your intuition and then have the courage to step in and follow through with all your heart without any expectations, life starts to create through you.

You begin to realize nothing is out of reach, everything is accessible. So long as it's true for you to create.

You can waste so much time and energy, running a million miles an hour, desperate for success in the hopes that you can finally outpace your demons. Only to realize that your resistance to following your truth has been the creator of them all along.

Listen to your intuition, follow its guidance and don't question it. No matter how crazy, irrational or silly it seems.

Because if you do, what you truly love will come to life.

As If By Magic.

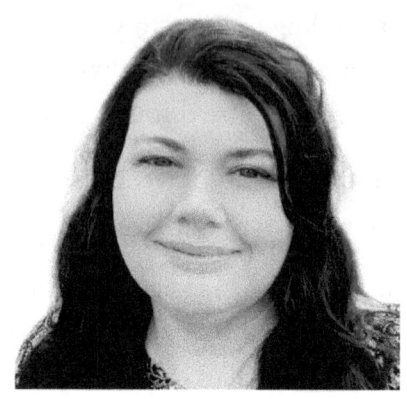

Jodie M Lavery

https://facebook.com/jodiemlavery2
https://www.instagram.com/jodie.m.lavery

Jodie's life is a shining example of the power of love, care, and creativity.

With a passion for writing that has only grown stronger with time, she has developed a deep love for both fiction and non-fiction.

As an Australian-based mother and grandmother. Jodie balances family responsibilities with her writing dreams, armed with two writing certificates and a developing short story.

Finding solace in nature, Jodie draws inspiration from being out in the great outdoors, camping and exploring.

When Jodie is not writing you will find her capturing the beauty of wildlife, flowers, and nature through photography.

Jodie's enduring commitment to both her family and her writing dreams is truly inspirational.

The Journey to Finding My Heart – From Darkness to Light

By Jodie M Lavery

I am unsure when I came to live within the walls of darkness, where the outside world kept spinning while I was hiding away, not wanting to be seen and oblivious to what was happening outside. Being in the darkness was like a bubble of protection, it was my comfort zone. It was a very lonely bubble, a complicated bubble no one could understand. It was not until the year 2020 that I became aware of how much I had sunk into that bubble of darkness. I was on my knees begging for anyone or anything to please clear the darkness I had fallen into and provide me the clarity I desperately needed. At the time, I was surrounded by a supportive partner, five grown gorgeous kids, a beautiful grandson, and a loving family. We had a stunning family home on the coast of Western Australia. Life was great, I was camping, exploring, going to the beach, and spending quality time with my loved ones. It sounded like the perfect life, but it was not. It did not matter what anyone or I did—the darkness was still there grasping me tightly, squeezing any hope inside me. I was suffocating, something was missing and I felt it deep within me. What I did know was that I was meant to do more with my life, but I was lost.

I became a Mum the year I turned 21, I was blessed with a little girl. Before I knew it, I was a mother of five children, 3 gorgeous boys and 2 beautiful girls, stuck in a marriage with a house we could not leave. The day did finally come when the children and I found the opportunity to escape the nightmare that was our life and went to live with my parents.

I became a carer for my oldest son the year he turned ten, I felt I was handed a certificate congratulating me for having a son with autism. It was not until he finished high school, we were granted assistance and support. I was in my second marriage then, living in a small country town, with my husband and five kids. During that time my mother sadly passed away, she was my best friend, and I spoke to her every day. My mother taught me many things, except how to live without her. Not long after my mother's passing, my husband and I decided to separate. This left me as a single Mum with two failed marriages and a diagnosis of social anxiety. The days seem to fly into weeks, weeks into months, and months into years.

I did find the courage to put myself out there again after 3 years of divorce. I asked my mother to please send me a loving, kind, supportive partner, a man whom I could spend the rest of my life with. My mother answered me and sent me just that. He was everything I asked my mother for. He stepped up, took on my five children, and treated them as his own.

As the years passed, two of our children left the nest to spread their wings, my partner and I were engaged, we celebrated the birth of our beautiful grandson, and we moved to the coast. I took up crocheting, jigsaw puzzles, word games, and watching movies. Anything to abolish the feeling inside and clear that familiar feeling of being in darkness. It would not budge, at this stage, I was destined to stay there.

I remember the first time I felt the darkness shift slightly; I was taking some photos on my phone. I felt so creative and inspired by taking photographs that my partner went out and bought me an SLR camera. The excitement I felt when I took that first photograph on a real camera was absolutely amazing. Somehow, I had this natural ability to photograph wildlife and flowers. From there, I went on and studied a Travel Writing Photography certificate, and every time I was behind that camera, something magical happened. I was transported to a place where I was at ease, feeling connected to what I was photographing, and the result led to amazing photos.

Later that year, my sister-in-law Tanya and I decided to go camping on our own. Camping was not new to me. I had been camping numerous times with my parents as a little girl and more recently with my partner. The thought of camping on our own scared me but excited me too. While we walked, we photographed and explored the camping area. I discovered a love of adventure and rekindled my love of camping and writing. Being out in nature, I found myself to be so inspired and motivated that it had shifted the darkness enough to allow a crack of the light through.

My sister-in-law and I continued to adventure more after that camping trip. My partner was working away and our children at home had all grown up and were now independent, so it allowed me more freedom to go. Even though the darkness disappeared a little bit more each camping trip, I still felt like something was missing. I was still feeling unbalanced, incomplete, anxious, fearful, and not living to my full potential. I felt greedy for wanting more out of life, what else could I need? What was I searching for? I was confused by these feelings, but I kept pushing them away, reminding myself I was being silly.

When I was not camping, or spending time with my loved ones, I found myself scrolling Facebook. It became my daily ritual, being distracted with post after post desperately searching for an answer, a sign, anything. I felt so alone on this journey, it seemed no one would understand the feelings I was dealing with inside me. It was a continuous battle of feeling so worthless, not good enough, not professional enough, not pretty enough, I just felt stuck. The only thing that made me truly happy and alive was venturing out, being one with nature, photographing, and spending time with my loved ones. I was always left wondering when and if things would change.

After endless months of scrolling Facebook, a video did grab my attention. It was a video of a lady, her name was Kelly, and she was standing with her horse and talking about an opportunity. It moved something in me and suddenly, I felt emotional inside. I heard a familiar voice within me that I had heard before, but I never paid attention to it. It said, "Say yes." I do not know what made me listen to this voice, maybe it was the video, or it could have been Kelly's words. I do not know; I just knew I had to discover more about this opportunity!

I reached out to Kelly and discovered the opportunity was more than an affiliate marketing opportunity, it contained an educational platform to learn everything I needed to know and a chance to work on personal development. Unfortunately, at that time, I could not afford the amount to begin the opportunity. I honestly did not know how or when I'd find the money to start the opportunity, it seemed impossible, but I knew I'd find it. I decided to stay within the free Facebook group Kelly invited me to and participate as much as possible.

The group led me to a special book, called *The Magic*. It contained daily practices that focused on gratitude. While practising gratitude in this book, I found magic for the first time. By the end of the book, it was obvious I was not only missing gratitude, but I was also missing magic in my life. Markedly, this has been the most transformational book I have ever read. The most memorable part of the book was Day 9 of The Magic, the daily practice was called Money Magnet. I was to take any unpaid bills I had, use gratitude's magical power, write across the unpaid bill, "Thank you for the money," and feel grateful for having the money to pay the bill whether or not I had it. We were camping at the time; I had no bill on me. So, I wrote a bill on a piece of paper for the amount I needed to join the opportunity and used that. I wrote "thank you for the money" across the bill with all my heart and so full of gratitude. We called it an early night due to setting off home early in the morning.

As soon as we came into phone service that next morning, a message popped up on my phone that I would receive a phone call from Centrelink shortly on. No caller ID. My first thought was what now? I waited anxiously for this phone call to come through. Finally, I thought,

I answered the call thinking it was bad news but to my surprise, the lady on the phone was explaining that they owed me money due to balancing the end of the financial year. I suddenly gasped as I heard her tell me how much they were depositing in my account, it was the exact amount I wrote on that bill the day before. My partner and I could not believe it! It was magical! This is the first time, well that I knew of that magic entered my life. I kept saying thank you to the universe all day. Most people I told put it down to coincidence, not me.

That next day, I joined the opportunity! I thoroughly enjoyed the twelve months or so I participated in the opportunity. I learned a lot about business, marketing, and most importantly, myself. I pushed myself out of my comfort zone numerous times and did things I never thought I could do. Unfortunately, in the end, I burnt myself out mentally. I felt I was doing all the right things but I just could not get the feeling of being fake, not good enough, not worthy enough out of mind. Every day I was feeling less aligned with the opportunity, and it left me feeling guilty for letting people down, even the universe.

A fellow member of that opportunity shared a post about a masterclass this lady was hosting. I had followed this lady named Theresa for a while. After attending the masterclass, Theresa reached out about a five-week program she felt would serve me. I instantly said yes as that familiar weird feeling inside me and that voice saying yes had returned. I did not know how it was going to help, somehow, I just knew.

In that five-week program, I felt a huge shift within me. Finally, I discovered that the weird thing I kept feeling inside me was my heart and that voice I heard saying yes was my inner voice. I continued to attend some of Theresa's other masterclasses she held throughout the year when I felt the call to participate.

I will always remember my first amazing experience working with Theresa, she introduced me to meditation, the land of plenty. I was sitting in silence, with my breath, I set the intention to clear the darkness, to show me what I am not allowing myself to see. As soon as I had entered the land of plenty, I heard the word 'write' very loud and clear, I could feel it in my heart. I thought weird, okay. Nothing else seemed to be coming through so I held on to the moment a little longer, I then heard the word 'empath.' I felt this strong sensation in my head. I sat with that sensation for a little, and a vision came to me. I was searching a boundary of shrubs. I asked myself, "What are you searching for?" The word 'confidence' flashed by, and I said, "Is that all I am looking for?" A clearing appeared like a tunnel. I was feeling a little scared, it looked dark inside. I told myself to have the confidence to walk through the tunnel, so I did.

As I reached the end of the tunnel, a beautiful beach came into view, I could see someone in the distance. I walked closer and as soon as it became clear who was standing there, my eyes filled with instant tears. It was my mother, she looked so beautiful. I said to my mum, "What are you doing here"? She said, "To tell you that you have many unique gifts and a big heart." I said, "Mum, what am I searching for?" She said, "Your heart, your purpose in life." I asked her, "What is my purpose?" She said, "Continue connecting and listening to that big heart of yours, it will guide you, share your heart with the world, and be of service." I said, "Serve who." Mum replied as she walked away, "Everyone, through your writing, your writing needs to be out in the world." It was the most beautiful moment; I did not want it to end. It was the first time I had a connection with my mum since she passed. She suddenly disappeared and I opened my eyes to tears rolling down my face. It was not only the first time I had a connection with my mum since she passed, but it was also the first time I felt a strong connection with my heart.

After this experience, I sat for a while thinking. In minutes, it came to me to start writing about my adventures and the places I had visited. I wrote about my travels to the Southwest, the Wheatbelt and the Peel area of Western Australia. It did not last long, all my writings are in a file on my laptop. I lost my confidence and hid the file deep away. So, with fear alongside the other things, I told myself about not being good enough, not worthy enough, etc. I retreated to the darkness, where I felt safe.

Two years had passed since I first felt the darkness shift and it was obvious my heart was not ready to give in. Once again, I heard that familiar voice, my inner voice, screaming at me. "Jodie! Apply, and you will be chosen for this!" Theresa was offering a year's scholarship to a program she had created. I was not considering applying for the scholarship as all those negative thoughts, which I now know are my Ego, were hammering my inner thoughts. Of course, my heart won and I applied. I never told anyone that I had the feeling I was going to be chosen, I did not know how I knew, I just knew. Just like magic, I was chosen. At that moment, I truly believed, in the universe, magic, and my inner voice.

My time on the scholarship changed my life dramatically, like never before. I was introduced to my superconscious, I had never heard of that word before, although, I learnt it is where my genius comes from. I knew I believed in magic, but I did not know magic is found in the unknown and that we do not need to know how something will happen for magic to happen. That's the power of magic. I quickly realised just how powerful of a human being I was. I created choices that led to the end result that I authentically desired. I could even live an inspired life, inspired by my genius and creativity by being me, my authentic self, and following my heart's desires.

For the first time, I was fully out of the darkness, participating in circles that Theresa held. This is where I discovered intuition and how strong it is. I always thought it was magical when things happened and I did not know how they happened, I just knew they would happen. I now have the awareness that was my intuition guiding me. I came to trust my intuition and listen to my heart, which led me to rediscover my love of writing again; I was now fully aware it was one of my natural abilities and was ready to share it with the world. I began writing inspirational and empowering posts on my Facebook. To my surprise, writing these posts came naturally to me with ease and flow. I believed I truly was talented. I felt so aligned, balanced, powerful, and seen.

Towards the end of my scholarship, I was introduced to a course that delved deeper into what I had been learning and practising in the program with Theresa. Leading with my heart and with inspired action, I entered the course. The training William Whitecloud had created was mind-blowing, it had a profound impact on me, evoking a deeper connection to my creative genius and my heart. During the course, I dug deep, it was uncomfortable, but I held the tension and played it fully out. In doing so I discovered more hidden beliefs I perceived as true about myself. I also found that deconstructing conflict quickly changed my relationship with conflict, it helped me hear what my unconscious was saying, taking the power out of it which allowed me to focus on my superconscious preference.

As soon as I finished the course, I felt so activated. I pulled out pieces of blank paper from the top drawer under my desk and started to write my first-ever short story, to my father's delight. My father has always believed since I was a little girl that I should write. He has had an idea for a story for so long, waiting for me to wake up to what he knew all along. After an hour of writing, I stopped, looked at my work, and thought, did I write this? Like magic, pages and pages of writing were lying there on the desk. Picking up the pages in my hands, I read each one. I found myself laughing, full of wonder and curiosity, about what would happen next.

This was an amazing time in my life, I felt grounded and fully connected to my heart. With courage and feeling ready. I surprised everyone and studied for my learner's test, I knew I'd pass with full marks, and the following week I did. I've never had my license, I always feared it, even sitting in the driver's seat with the engine off frightened me. I always felt hopeless, anxious, and not smart enough to drive. After passing my learner's, I remember just sitting in the driver's seat, my ego was there, I acknowledged it and it was welcomed to stay, as long as it did not voice its opinion.

Driving for the first time, I felt on top of the world, I had conquered a major fear I had held on to for way too long. I always thought it would be one fear I'd never overcome. It reminded me that my thoughts and feelings are not real, they are only what I perceive as real. Within a few weeks of having my learner's, I confidently drove into the city and even to the country to my father's place.

I honestly thought life could not be any better. I was camping, hiking and exploring as much as possible. I was fully in my genius, writing, photographing, and driving when I could. Everything just kept falling into place like magic.

I became so engrossed in writing the short story I had started that I had pushed aside all I had learned and practised within the scholarship and the course I attended. Life got in the way, and slowly, day by day, I crept away from everything back into that place I had known so well—the darkness. I was so disconnected from my heart, my greatness, and myself. I went back to hanging out with my ego. The only thing I did continue was camping, exploring, and hiking. Being out in nature camping was the only time I felt connected to my heart enough for the ego to take a backseat. I would feel so inspired and back in my genius every time I was out in nature. As soon as I returned home, I went back into the darkness with my ego. It was an ongoing saga.

This pattern led me to throw myself into every marketing opportunity anyone flashed at me like a new shiny object. Every single opportunity I started on a high, with me putting 100 percent of my time, money, and energy into it. I never recruited anyone; I did not make much money at all. After boredom set in, I would drop that opportunity and move on to the next. I was on a hamster wheel of affiliate marketing. It was never-ending. I did hear my inner voice talking to me, loud and clear but I continued to ignore it. My heart was in pieces, screaming at me as I was no longer connected to it. I knew deep down this was not my path, not my calling, not my why, and not what my heart desired. Still, I continued to take action with every single opportunity, it was not inspired action, it was half-hearted. That is why I never had the results I wanted.

What I truly wanted was to return to when I felt aligned with my heart, living with inspired action and being in my genius but I did not know how to get back there. I began meditating again and practising gratitude. I spent days sitting quietly with my breath to ground myself. I went back to writing inspiring and empowering posts on Facebook, sprinkling love from my heart to everyone. I went back and reread everything I had learned in the past. Last of all, I answered my heart's desire. I remembered my why and began writing my short story again, listening to my inner voice and following my heart. I still felt full of fear, it was stopping me from my true potential. I knew what I feared, but I did not know how to move past it.

At the end of last year my partner came home from Fly in, Fly out extremely ill, at one point I thought I was going to lose him. He was in and out of the hospital for a few months before he came well. This was a major wake-up call for me, I remember sitting there beside his hospital bed one day and thinking that life is so short, why am I spending it hiding in the darkness afraid? I made a promise right then and there to my heart and to the universe. If an opportunity came by authentically, I would get to the bottom of my fear and have my writing out into the universe before the end of the year.

The universe listened; it took me up on this challenge as I knew it would. Months later a friend of mine Jo, with whom I had spent time in the past in masterclasses, circles, and with her coaching, had shared a workshop she was holding about turning your fear into fuel. I signed up immediately, I knew this was a sign from the universe after all I did promise to take action. I looked forward to the workshop as I knew I was full of fear and was over it. I wanted to rid myself of it and stop it from consuming me. Fear was keeping me from many things, but more importantly, my potential.

In the masterclass, Jo uncovered a lot about fear, that I had never heard before. She taught us the process of writing to identify, reframe, and release fear. By the end of the workshop, I was excited to get started. I was more than ready to identify the fears within me, and finally release them. The second I started; my ego did make an appearance. I began telling myself I had already done a yearly scholarship, and went through an extensive course and still here I am fearful. How would this help? I stopped myself and said, "No ego, not today."

I found the writing process hard, confronting, and emotional. However, as soon as I established all the fears, it instantly hit me. I was responsible! All this time, I was responsible. I had created these fears within me, I believed the fears and I allowed myself to be consumed by them all. Those fears I created within me defined the outcome of my life, no wonder I kept running back into darkness. During that last part of the process after acknowledging the fears, it was overwhelmingly clear that since I created them, I could release them. After releasing the fears, I felt a huge weight lifted, it was such an intense moment.

Now I was free, free of fear to pursue my true purpose, my ultimate passion and live an inspired life. I find it hard to put into words how powerful this process was. Though, personally I feel the true power is in the writing. To go all in, be raw, and allow it all to flow out until it flows no more. It's an amazing feeling after all these years of having fear and now they are deleted just by identifying, reframing, and releasing the fear. It is truly astounding.

The next day, Jo checked in with me to see how I was feeling after yesterday's workshop. She mentioned that she had suggested my name to her friend, who was collaborating on a book. Instantly, I knew this was the universe putting me to the test, for the second part of my promise. I booked a session with Jo around resistance. It was time. Yes, my fears were gone but I still had resistance. The session ended up being very transformational for me. It led me to get to the bottom for once and all about my resistance and what was holding me at bay for all these years. Reaching the bottom was not an easy journey, with lots of resistance from me. With Jo's guidance, I reached the answers I had been seeking for so long. It landed with so much sense. I had the most massive cry after the session as I knew it was completely released. I will forever be so grateful for Jo's guidance.

Since that session, I have been reborn, that is exactly what it feels like. I am authentically aligned more than ever with my true nature and purpose. I am fully in tune with my heart and my life feels balanced. I am free from fear, resistance, and all the self-talk I told myself and believed for so long. Honestly, it feels like I have walked through a door from the past, and stepped into the now, grounded and ready to create magic through my creative spirit.

This led me to enter that short story I had been writing for so long and finished in a writing competition I had known about for many years. The competition advertisement has been magically popping up in places frequently, nudging me to enter. I did not hesitate at all. I just submitted it.

Of late, I have done things I never dreamed of doing or had the opportunity to do. I am so grateful for everyone who has been a part of this journey to finding my heart. It might have taken me forty-seven years, but I can say, I no longer fear being out in the light and being seen for the beautiful, authentic, big-hearted magical genius I am.

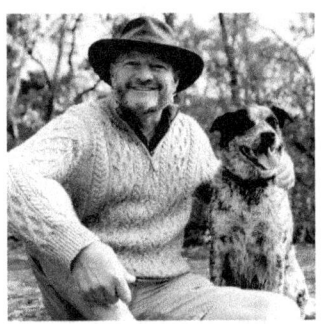

Guy Thornycroft

The Guy To Know Pty Ltd
Director

https://www.linkedin.com/in/guy-thornycroft/
https://www.facebook.com/profile.php?id=100063594606203
https://www.instagram.com/guytheguytoknow/
https://www.theguytoknow.com/

Guy was born and raised in Zimbabwe, attended Rhodes University in South Africa, learned financial planning in Scotland and now lives in Australia with his wife, Fiona and four children. He plays the Oboe and Highland Bagpipes and loves free diving.

Professionally, Guy has worked extensively with financial planners, accountants, lawyers and small-business owners in support, consulting and coaching roles. He presents at conferences, worked on numerous committees, runs his own company and directed others.

Guy teaches couples and individuals, a collection of powerful tools and shares knowledge with people who are ready to be inspired and grow. His objective is self aware, self accountable clients who take action to define and create the life they dream of.

His mission is to work with clients over the years of their growth and discovery, helping them return to their natural whole, creative and powerful state, as commanders of their own lives.

A Dilemma of Cost

By Guy Thornycroft

The END.

Failure was something I couldn't face, but was undeniably eating me up from the inside like a parasite in my heart. I was not happy, and despite my best efforts, I couldn't see change happening any time soon. I was in a rut, but I scarcely knew it, for failure was shameful and shame was unthinkable; to be denied at all costs.

It certainly wasn't my fault, I told myself, just some unfortunate twists of fate that had led me to this exhausting and impossible state of affairs. I had no idea that my life was about to change so deeply. I'd always smirked at the thought that we learn from history but looking back there was plenty I may have noticed if I'd cared to look.

If you ever saw the film *Dead Poet Society* with Robin Williams, you'd know the type of boys-only private boarding school, I grew up in. To cry was weakness and invited merciless ridicule. Failure was not tolerated and was swiftly punished. A Victorian approach to toughen boys up and fill their heads with 'Crown and Country' that was well backed up by my grandparents in school holidays. Wonderful, well-meaning people but children were to be seen and not heard. So, success and achievement were my means of survival. It all came down to how well I played cricket or tennis and winning swimming or shooting competitions helped. In my mind, I had to win to be loved and accepted. The problem was I didn't feel I was winning anymore! How had it come to this?

After finishing university in South Africa, Fiona and I went to find a place to live in the world. Africa was looking unstable and so we began what was meant to be a three-year world tour to find a place to nest. Those were carefree and happy days of working a little and playing a great deal. Winchester, UK, was our first base, from which we explored the South of England and much of Wales. Cash jobs were easy and, as an engaged couple, life was a loving adventure.

That all changed when we moved our base to Scotland. Jobs were scarcer and an affordable place to live harder to find and it was not long before I found myself, by chance, of course, in full-time work as a hotel manager working 65–70 hours a week. I justified it as a career opportunity and good for the CV. It made me feel I was important and in demand. In truth, I was a slave and naively being taken advantage of. At work, I was all too ready to please, and when at home exhausted.

It was always our plan to get married and so we did. I didn't imagine it would change us that much and life would continue as a loving couple. In truth, it shouldn't have, but for me, it massively increased the self-imposed pressure to perform. It layered on obligations that I assumed came with being a husband.

I'll always be grateful for the worst night I had at the hotel. A new General Manager (GM) had lost a hotel he managed to fire in Aviemore and was, as a result, super alert to that risk. Our fire alarms were set to their highest sensitivity and a few weeks did not include a full evacuation when the steam from a hot shower set off a corridor alarm or a staff member smoked too close to a fire exit. There were a few other unsavoury characteristics of this GM. He was short, balding, and middle-aged and thought it was fun to pinch the bums of the young barmaids and restaurant staff. He had a string of failed marriages and I suspect a drinking problem. He was strict and demanding and I have no doubt he knew how to run a hotel, but he was socially repugnant.

On the night in question, I was significantly understaffed for a Wedding Party of 300 from Glasgow. They had been bussed in and as they arrived had stormed the bar. Instantly they were 10 deep and the guests at the front realising it would take ages to get a second round of drinks were ordering 3 rounds at a time. We ran out of glasses and then ran out of beer and that was the start of the trouble. My casual bar staff started leaving under the pressure of being shouted at and abused. The kitchen needed me to run the event. The bar staff needed me to change kegs and find more glasses. The reception desk needed me to deal with unhappy guests and I didn't want to be there at all. The night was just starting.

The first fire alarm went off at 9pm. A drunk and disgruntled wedding guest held a cigarette lighter to a sensor. Reception phones lit up with guests asking if it was a drill; the fire brigade sirens letting them know it was not; and the staff following their emergency routine. The first full evacuation and roll call went off faultlessly and I thanked the fire brigade for their quick response. I thanked the guests for their understanding, and I thanked the staff for their efficiency in handing out blankets and printing off guest lists.

Around 10pm I had a face-off with the best man who was armed with a screwdriver and wanted to introduce it to my face for ruining his friend's wedding. Shortly after I had dealt with him, the fire alarms went off again. I never worked out how they were set off but I knew well enough who was responsible. My hotel guests were less understanding, the fire brigade less friendly and my staff a little less good-natured. I wasn't having such a great time myself.

By 11pm I had evacuated the whole hotel for the third time. This time was more serious. A certain wedding guest had pulled a wash basin in the gents off the wall. The high-pressure hot water tap was shooting a jet of steaming hot water up into the ceiling above, collapsing it and the water was flooding the floor below, bringing that ceiling down too. The water was too hot to duck under to get to the safety tap. I'd had enough. I called the police for backup and refused to let the wedding guests back in. Between the bitterly complaining hotel guests and the angry drunk wedding party, I was not feeling loved.

I didn't get much sleep but knew I had to be at the reception for the checkout of disgruntled guests. That over, I faced up to the GM for a debrief. I felt like such a failure. I sat in silence waiting for him to fire me. He shuffled a pile of paper in front of him and then smiled at me. When he spoke, it was not what I was expecting. He was impressed. He had received congratulations for my actions from the fire brigade. He had spoken to the police and received a glowing report about my decisions and leadership. He had spoken to the staff and was impressed by what they said. I should be proud. I'd done well. Somewhere in all this nightmare, there appeared a glimmer of hope and then the words that changed everything: "If you keep this up, you will be GM, just like me!" I was going to end up just like him!

It dawned on me that if I stayed in the hotel game, I would end up 'just like him'. My resignation was in by the end of the week.

By chance, an older family friend, Peter, was looking for a Practice Manager for his Financial Planning business and was delighted I could fill the position. I spent the next two years training to be an adviser and dreaming of making more money. I needed it as we bought our first house, Fiona landed a scholarship to do a Doctorate and our first child arrived. I enjoyed my work and felt appreciated, useful, and an important part of its success. The office was dog friendly and at lunch, we would take our dogs to a park and train them to fetch or sit and wait. On weekends, we often shot clay pigeons or went fly fishing together. Peter and I were good friends, but when he suggested it was time to retire and I was his succession plan, I was terrified. It was all very well working under him but not without his wisdom and guidance!

By chance, I discovered the company that provided the financial planning software we used was expanding into Australia and was looking for someone who knew it well enough to sell it there for them. Prestwood Software was owned and run by a very well-regarded and internationally recognised man who was happy to take me on and assisted greatly with our move to Gosford, New South Wales, Australia.

It was an exciting move. Away from the cold and wet of Scotland to the heat and dust of Australia. Fiona just managed to finish her Doctorate a few days before we left and was heavily pregnant with our second child when we landed. The first night in Australia I looked up at the stars and felt waves of homesickness because, after 5 years in the Northern Hemisphere, I was seeing stars I recognised from Africa! I had everything to look forward to and a business to build under the guidance of powerful men. I worked hard to impress them and earn enough money to buy our own home and just enough to provide for two and then three children. I could have been happy but I wasn't.

Have you ever had the wrong key in your hand that went into the lock but no matter how you jiggle it and turn it, it won't turn or open the lock? I felt like that key. I was on the road 3 weeks out of 4 visiting financial planners around the country and clocking up the frequent flyer points. I was back to working long hours and feeling that I was missing out on time with my family, but it was my duty to provide so I was driven on to succeed. Only, I just didn't fit into the industry. It wasn't my fault, of course, just that I wasn't Australian enough perhaps. Maybe it was because the competition had more money to spend on their marketing. Despite my passion to make a difference, I was having little impact on a profession entrenched in their ivory towers and happy with the easy money they were making. I felt I wasn't trying hard enough, and I certainly didn't feel good enough, but the show had to go on.

So, there I was with three children, a large mortgage, in a job that was not taking off fast enough for me to feel I was winning and no idea of how to change any of it. Well, it is not fair to say I had no idea because there were hints there was an easier way to live life playing in my mind, almost at my fingertips and on the tip of my tongue but frustratingly out of my reach, like dreams that fade when you focus on them. Impossible to articulate but with growing intensity I was noticing contradictions. There were suggestions of magic that were gently landing on my awareness. What were these whispers of magic?

For example, have you ever noticed that with some jars, the harder you grip the lid, the tighter it grips to the jar making it increasingly harder to open? Sometimes you have to put less grip into the twist and replace it with the illogical downward pressure that might be seen as holding the lid more firmly on, rather than helping remove it. Or have you ever heard of over-brushing your teeth? In an attempt to have the cleanest most well-kept teeth, you can actually harm them and remove the enamel, push back the gums and expose them to faster decay! I'd noticed that the more urgently I needed to get somewhere on time, the slower the traffic and the more red lights there seemed to be. The more I needed a certain card to win, the lower the chance of it turning up. The more my children tried to hide the truth from someone, the guiltier they came across. I could hit any number on a dart board when it was just me in the garage, but as soon as I was showing off and trying to impress someone, mysteriously the darts turned on their magical board-avoidance systems. It was as if my wanting something badly rendered it unattainable and it led to some very strange behaviour of pretending disinterest and trying to attain by stealth. Of never asking for what I wanted directly and always feeling disappointed by my Christmas Gifts. I blamed others for my misery. After all, if they only knew me well enough or cared enough, they would just know what I wanted. To me, asking for what I wanted cheapened the value of receiving it at best or prevented me from having it at all.

By chance, when the pressure was at its highest, I was given a book for Christmas in 2005 by a client that changed my life forever. It was *The Magician's Way* by William Whitecloud and I read it from cover to cover riveted by its revelations. In it, he explained every concept that had been hovering at the edge of my mind and I was so excited. I finished the book on a Wednesday afternoon and immediately found a phone number to call this mysterious man who seemed to be so aligned with what I had been finding out for myself.

The call was answered by Claire Scott-Lister, his assistant, who let me know I had just missed him, but there was a course he was running. I didn't hesitate and asked her to sign me up. I wouldn't miss it for the world. Claire was a bit taken aback.

"But I haven't told you how much it is," she said.

"I don't care, I'm coming!" I replied enthusiastically

"But you don't know how long it is either," she countered.

"OK," I conceded, *"tell me all about it."*

Claire went on to tell me it was $8,000 for the course plus flights, meals and accommodation. All up around $10,000 for a yearlong training.

That stopped me in my tracks. One weekend away each month for nearly a year! I was hardly home as it was and $10 grand? We were up to our necks in the house debt and had forgotten what the word savings meant. What really scared me was the thought of talking to Fiona about it! *"Hey, you know, I'm hardly ever home and we have no money to spare but..."* I could imagine all too well how that conversation was going to end!

I asked Claire to give me 48 hours to work it out. I knew in my heart I wanted to be on that course. I just couldn't see how to make it happen. What a dilemma! I said nothing to Fiona that night and, as usual, was at work at 8am Thursday morning. On my way to my desk, I passed our Managing Director, Ian, and we greeted each other warmly, but a few paces past me he turned and called me back, having just remembered a conversation he had the night before with the Group Director in the UK.

"Guy," he said. *"We notice you have not done any training in the last three years and we think you should be learning something. Do you have anything in mind that you could do?"*

I couldn't believe what I was hearing, but without hesitation replied, *"Well, there is this course I'm looking at..."*

"Great", he said. *"Book it in!"*

"But I haven't told you how much it is," I stammered

"I don't care," he replied. *"If you think it will be of value, do it!"*

"But you don't know how long it is either," I countered.

"That's not my concern, Guy," Ian said over his shoulder, already heading off.

I know Claire was more than a little surprised to get my call, but I couldn't have been happier. I think if I'd known what I was letting myself in for, I would have never made that call! Thus, it was that from January 2006, once a month, I would fly from Sydney to The Gold Coast and with a dozen others catch a minibus for the two-hour drive to the training venue. The accommodation was a single large room for the men with matrasses on the floor and the hall was packed with about 120 attendees, arranged into teams. I'm still close friends with many of my team, The Wolves.

Having never done any creative or self-development work, I was in the deep end with no option but to try and stay afloat. My arrogant self-important nature had me fighting from the start and there were times like the first intuitive ego reading that remains an embarrassment. For that particular exercise, we were broken into groups of four strangers, and being excited and expectant, I volunteered to be the first read. I made my statement and sat back ready to be praised, but of course, this was a reading about my beliefs and egoic strategies and what followed was 15 minutes of the most humiliating and devastating dressing down I could imagine. I sat there with tears running down my face (embarrassing enough!) as the three women saw right through my bravado to my most intimate secrets and calmly told me I was not good enough, unworthy and incapable. The most painful cut was heartlessly telling me that without a powerful male role model to copy, I believed I was nothing. It was my worst nightmare and just set to get worse.

When the ordeal was finally over, they cheerfully said it was my turn to do it to them! I flatly refused! In front of 120 people, I stood up and loudly accused William of fostering bullying and ridicule and declaring that I would have nothing more to do with it. I stormed out of the hall, my mind in a turmoil of shame and confusion. It took William quite some time to calm me down and explain what was happening to me and longer to convince me to return, my pride in tatters. It didn't kill me but there were times I wished the ground would swallow me up.

Each month brought its own challenges and steep learning but as the months progressed, I found the most exciting and extraordinary thing and that was the taming of my emotions; a falling away of my pretence; a waking up to my certainty, confidence, and creativity. I was responding less and actively engaging more. Importantly, I learned to deal with conflict and calmly speak my truth. I began to believe in magic and critically learned the difference between creative tension and stress and how to depower the latter and leverage the former to bring about what I wanted. I was waking up to a power I had suspected but never been able to call on.

Please don't imagine I left that year a master! Far from it, but in the years to follow that was to change utterly and this is how it happened.

Applying the knowledge I had learned, I worked smarter and made considerably more sales. I joined committees and boards and established myself as an authority. I moved the company past breakeven and we began to attract interest from the bigger players. I was still working hard and while I had a great deal of discretion. there was still a managing director and Group Owner to please, but I was enjoying the work more. I was beginning to see some great potential and dreaming of making considerably more money.

One memorable occasion illustrates how much I was changed by the work. I didn't feel as if I were any different, but my behaviour sure was. I flew to Brisbane for an awards night. I was staying in a B&B and caught the bus to the venue. I was dressed in my tuxedo and it was very cold. There were road works and the bus driver had to take a detour between heavy concrete blocks for 100m. At the end of the diversion, the gap that had been left for her to turn out of was too narrow to manoeuvre the bus through. We were stuck! She radioed for help and was informed they would send someone out, but it would be an hour or more before they could put a team together. She announced the news to the bus and because of protocol couldn't open the door to let us out! There was a lot of anger and she was genuinely afraid and embarrassed. I could feel the familiar resentment, anger and twinge of fear. After all, I was meant to be at a smart dinner and now I was going to be late. It was going to cost me a great deal and the bus company would be hearing my complaint. A sense of powerlessness of being stuck and not being able to do anything about it. But on this occasion, I wasn't buying into the way it was. I found myself wondering what the bus driver was going through. I made my way to the front of the bus and started talking to her about her job and how long she had been driving for. She shared the current fear the drivers were experiencing on the back of one of them being sued. She didn't dare do anything that might be outside of the rules. I could see her calming down and feeling understood. I could feel she was glad to have one passenger on her side. That trust built as we talked some more. After 20 minutes the office radioed to say it would be another two hours wait. I saw her tense to tell the passengers and had an inspiration. I leant in and hatched a plan in which I would get off the bus and direct her through a multi-point turn to get back onto the road and no one need know how she had done it! To see the look of relief in her eyes that she didn't have to give the passengers more bad news was amazing and that's what we did. I took control of the traffic and helped her shuffle that bus back and forward until it slipped through the small gap and then leapt back on board. By then the whole bus was aware of what we were doing and she announced that I had saved them two hours further delay. The bus erupted into applause and shouts of congratulations to her for having saved the day. It turned from an angry mob to a party bus. Everyone talking excitedly to each other and much back slapping and hand shaking on my way back to my seat. Who was this new me? I liked them!

Then in 2010, out of the blue, I received a redundancy. The software company was given a golden opportunity to capture most of the English market and to do that it needed to close its international operations. 10 years of slog was at an end and while I should have been shocked and worried, my whole world opened up. It was almost a relief. I took three months off to consider my options and recover. I had my first taste of real freedom having time with our now four children. I never wanted to go back to working for a master again. I wanted to be my own boss.

I had this grand plan and with the redundancy money I launched my own business. Spending thousands on marketing and sales materials, I utterly failed to cover my cost. Despite everyone I spoke to telling me what a great idea it was. Despite all the free talks and promotions I ran. Despite following the advice of every guru I went to...wait! Why was I still trying to follow gurus? It was only at this point I saw the recurring pattern. Not just finding a powerful man to study under but the actions I was taking each time to impress. The same actions lead to the same results and dissatisfaction. It was like a blindfold had been taken off and the world had changed from grey to a kaleidoscope of opportunity.

I reinvented my business and changed its name. I no longer needed to copy and follow but became 'The Guy to Know'. It was my turn at the top and I was ready to take up that calling. As if by magic, opportunities came consistently and in a few short years, I was running a highly profitable business, working from home and taking four-day weekends every fortnight. It feels like I'm no longer looking for a light in the dark, but shining my own light and drawing others to me, only to send them out again shining theirs. I believe we all have it within ourselves to shine and sometimes it just takes someone to remind us. It's a beautiful world filled with more treasures and adventures than I could hope to experience in a lifetime. I'm hell-bent on trying to fit in as many as I can.

The BEGINNING

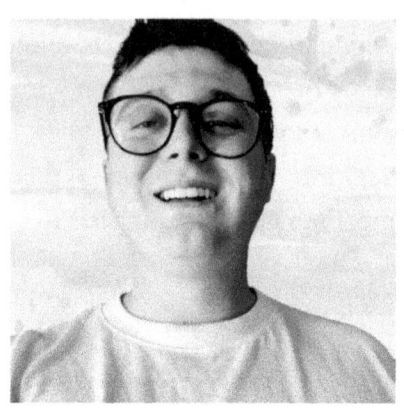

Austin Florek

Life Coach

https://www.facebook.com/austin.florek.7
https://www.instagram.com/toofarout1/
https://www.youtube.com/@ToofaroutTV
https://asteroidaustin.gumroad.com/

Austin Florek, based in Ohio, USA, is a transformational life coach with a powerful personal story. Growing up in poverty and a fractured home, he battled drug addiction before embarking on a journey of redemption and self-discovery. Today, Austin channels his past struggles into a mission of service, aiming to positively impact the world and future generations of his family. His drive to effect meaningful change reflects a deep commitment to personal growth and empowerment, inspiring others to overcome adversity and achieve their fullest potential. Through his work as a coach and mentor, Austin embodies resilience and hope, dedicated to creating a brighter, more compassionate world for all.

For free content from Austin, Connect with him on YouTube or Facebook!

Divine Intuition

By Austin Florek

Growing up bouncing between homes, Mom and Dad were never married. They did their best to love me, with the tools they had, although I wasn't willing to recognize that for the longest time. I felt alone, unseen, and unloved. These feelings caused problems for me, as I didn't know where they were coming from, and I wasn't willing to look. I spent my childhood learning how to and successfully running away from my feelings. I thought they were bad, and because they were inside me, I was bad. I began to act out in school, seeking attention wherever I could get it from, and this normally ended up in me getting in trouble, which just reinforced the "bad" feelings I felt inside. Soon, I started to mask my emotions by using drugs and alcohol. The first time I tried them, I was hooked.

My life quickly started to spiral out of control. In middle school, I began smoking marijuana and taking pills. Before I graduated high school, I was using heroin on most days. I would steal from you, lie to you, and somehow make it your fault that I did any of it. When I couldn't have what I wanted, I would isolate myself, cry, and complain, and the only thing I could focus on was not having the drugs I was withdrawing from. My existence was miserable, and my actions were only making it worse. The justice system took an interest in me after my parents turned me in to the police for my drug use. Their intentions were to help me, but I took it the wrong way and now saw my parents as the enemy. I started isolating more, running away, and looking at everything outside of me as the problem of why I felt and acted this way.

Although my parents turned my stuff in to the police station, and I got into legal trouble and was put on probation, it didn't stop me from using drugs to escape. This started to bring me consequences I didn't like, in the form of going to treatment centers, Alcoholics Anonymous meetings, more strict probation, and going to jail. I became so sick of everything in my life and environment that a girlfriend and I decided to run away across the country. I drove across the whole United States of America with no driver's license, no shoes on, and a felony warrant for my arrest. I was scared and I was running away, not knowing that no matter where I went, there I was! I continued to cause problems for myself and anyone around me. While in California, at a hotel for the evening, I realized my girlfriend at the time was in a different hotel room with another guy and had left me alone for the night. This crushed me and when she did finally return to our room, I told her it was time for us to end it and we were going back home. Once we arrived home, I was found by the police of my town and put into jail for a year. Even in jail, I found ways to get into trouble and was locked down because of it. This is the pattern that went on for a while until I started realizing that the things that were happening in my life were not always a result of someone else. Someone reminded me that I was the common denominator in all of my problems. I started to investigate my life, and while thinking back I realized that of all the "problems" in my life— there I was, the one causing it. The pattern became too obvious to miss, but too painful to admit. I continued to use drugs and alcohol to cover up the pain of this new realization, but something had changed. I knew too much to go on living my old way, and although it was hard to look at, I started making little changes. Little by little, I started to accept the way I was living wasn't going to get me anywhere and that I needed to do something different.

One day, after having this realization and knowing something changed inside of me, I found myself being angry and aggressive towards my child and my dog. This time I was able to see myself for what I was being in that moment. Instantly, I turned inward, knowing that something wasn't right. I couldn't figure out what was wrong with me. Have I been acting this way for a long time? Why am I being so cruel? How did I become so angry? Right around this same time, I was introduced to my first spiritual teacher on YouTube. Although I had no idea what I was doing, I prayed for the first time. I prayed to God for guidance and had my first spiritual experience, resulting in my spiritual awakening.

The only things that changed were inside of me. A place I have never visited on purpose, as I was committed to running away from my feelings at any cost. My mind had been on autopilot, always looking for ways to run from my emotions, and I realized that I had to go outside of my current frame of mind if I was going to make any change. I started to see the world differently, seeing more possibilities than ever; although, not sure how to take action on it. I began to explore more about the topics of spirituality and consciousness. Everything was so confusing. It felt like my world was flipped upside down, and although it was painful, I kept going. It was intriguing to see a new way of life and discover why things happened. There was new meaning in life as I started to look at the world through the eyes of love.

As I grew in my journey, I learned about how the mind works, and that mine had been running on autopilot based on the way I thought I should be from being taught by my family. Certain traditions, expectations, thought patterns, and beliefs were passed on to me like hand-me-downs, and since I had no idea what was what, I just took these beliefs on as my own. This meant that I was thinking, feeling, and acting like the other people in my family and environment without even knowing it. I wasn't being myself, I was being who I thought I should be based on their expectations. This led me to be very uncomfortable in my own skin because who was inside wasn't really me. I would act in strange ways, foreign to my heart and soul's true calling, seeking validation from others because I wasn't truly happy with myself.

During this awakening process, I started seeing things for how they truly were. I started seeing people for who they truly were. It was obvious to me that I had recently been living a big lie and the people around me were in on it. Nobody was being their true selves, we were all just pretending to be and act in a certain way because that is what is socially acceptable. Most of the conversations I found myself in were not authentic, instead, they were about putting someone else down so we could feel superior. I also learned what it meant to be empathic, that I could sense other people's emotions. This was the beginning of my intuitive abilities coming online. This heightened sense of empathy was used as a tool to feel someone else's emotions and make sure that they were having a good time or that I wasn't getting on their bad side. I developed this ability to ensure that I was a top-level people pleaser. I knew that if I could get on your good side, you wouldn't have anything against me and that maybe I could get what I wanted from you. I learned this out of fear. Because I was insecure, I didn't trust myself or my abilities. (How could I when I didn't truly know myself?) I would give my power and energy away to someone else so that they could take care of me.

A big example of this in my life, was when I realized the relationship I was in with my son's mother, was a codependent relationship. I was a "stay-at-home dad" at the time, while still addicted to using drugs to escape. She worked full-time and took care of all the bills. I never developed the confidence to earn my own money because I was afraid to take charge of my life. She didn't feel worthy unless she was providing for someone. Since I wasn't working and didn't have my own money, I began to feel trapped in the relationship and the house. When she would come home from work, I would give her all my love and affection in hopes that she would take us somewhere or be willing to spend her money on us to do something we could all enjoy. This was just another way for me to escape my emotions. It gave her a sense of power over me and I was okay with it because I felt powerless over myself. When I woke up to how this was playing out, I started to detach my energy from the situation. This was a hard thing for me because I had to take control of my own life, earn my own money, and think for myself. I had to become who I wasn't, and I had to do it alone.

As I started to detach my energy, I woke up a sleeping giant. The first experience of me claiming my power back was met with resistance. All of the relationships I had in life were based on a certain energy dynamic of me giving away my power in return for something. I let others control my mind for so long and had no idea it was happening. When I went to talk to someone else about my relationship situation, I was revealing to them that I was becoming more sovereign and they also didn't like it. Whether conscious of it or not, my friends and family started to see me as their competition. I was the one who wanted to change and see things for how they actually were. I wanted to grow and become who I never thought I could be. I was revealing to my friends and family the flaws in our relationships. I was now exposing the codependent behaviors that were present within the family, which is a huge disruption to someone who would rather stay asleep in the matrix. I found that people would rather live the way they have been living, even if it's causing harm to themselves or others because it's comfortable. To move into the unknown is uncomfortable and can bring up fear in an individual, making them resistant to change.

In November 2022, my father passed away from Lou Gehrig's Disease. This was a hard thing for the family, to watch a loved one suffer before leaving earth. It was a dramatic build-up to his final night, during a Scorpio Full moon. I remember falling asleep that night thinking about our last visit together, he couldn't talk so he spoke to me by focusing his eyesight onto a keyboard and it spoke for him. The next morning I woke up to a text that he had passed away, and immediately, without effort, I imagined feeling for him. I could sense his energy, it felt like he was flying around me with so much joy and enthusiasm. I couldn't help but feel a euphoric sensation come over me, and I knew at that moment he was happy and free. A few days after his passing, I was doing Kundalini Breathwork and had an experience I'll never forget. I started having flashes of memories and ideas that were all a synchronization of my life, and I could feel my dad's energy present. I was finally able to see how all the happenings in my life were orchestrating a bigger plan, and I knew which direction I would be going. I could feel my dad on the other side, blessing me with his presence and willingness to help. I could also see things I no longer wanted to be a part of. As this awakening unfolded, I was eager to share about it because it was exciting for me. When I shared these things with my family, a lot of them couldn't understand. I don't blame them for not understanding, but this definitely contributed to a feeling of loneliness and confusion. I could feel myself moving in new directions and away from what was no longer aligned.

The more I attempted to separate myself from these energies, the more I understood their grip on me. I had been keeping myself in this state, just like everyone else was because I was afraid to see the truth. Looking at the truth can sometimes be a hard thing to do, but a very rewarding process. This is when I chose to forgive myself and others for the way we had been acting. I chose to forgive others for allowing themselves to take advantage of me, and I chose to forgive myself for taking advantage of other people. I also chose to forgive myself for letting others treat me this way. Although it wasn't my fault that this happened, it was my responsibility to fix it. I also couldn't place the blame on anyone else because, of course, they were only doing what they thought was best with what tools they had available to them. These thought patterns and traditions have been passed down from generation to generation because nobody has put a stop to them. I may have come from a toxic family environment, but that doesn't mean a toxic family environment has to come from me.

It felt like a lot of people didn't understand what was happening to me. I was going through these changes, I was doing lots of research, and acting in a totally different manner than I had been. I was pulling away from my family and friends, which led to isolation and them wondering where my energy was. I would spend hours at a time watching YouTube videos about Spiritual Awakening and Tarot readings, and listening to audiobooks on the subjects that interested me. The things I thought about and talked about changed drastically, and I started to give people advice where I used to ask for advice. The people around me didn't like this because they were used to me leaning on them. Now that I was becoming the power in my own life, I didn't seek these people out anymore, and I could feel that they were starting to become resentful. It was obvious that I was changing and I had found a higher power in my life that was leading me towards a new opinion of myself, others, and life. I was becoming a new and empowered version of myself by directly disobeying the systems I had relied upon so much. The control systems within my family were one of the hardest things to overcome because I was conditioned to think I needed them and must accept them no matter how they acted. While becoming a new version of myself, I stopped accepting behavior that I thought was inappropriate in my life. I had to part ways with friends and separate myself from family members. It was clear that I was on a new path and trajectory that nobody in my life at the time had ever considered, or attempted to take on. I was dancing to the beat of my own drum, and I stood out.

Around this time, an ad for William Whitecloud's program "Create Your Destiny" appeared before me on the internet. The program called to me so loud, I immediately signed up. I still wasn't working and was battling my addiction, so when I saw that the program was free, I was so excited. I took the course and developed my first set of choices. These are like personal affirmations that direct our minds to focus on what our heart desires to create. Because I wasn't working, I couldn't move forward with the curriculum at that time. The course was exactly what I needed to get hope back into my life, I could finally set a new direction towards what truly aligned in my soul. This encouraged me to start making bigger changes. I began making my own YouTube videos discussing everything I learned through the last couple of years of rigorous study. My values started to change. Instead of wanting to run and hide from this emerging truth within, I decided to face it in a new direction, now I wanted to clear up my legal issues and clean out more of the bad feelings I was holding onto. I desired to get sober for the first time in my life. More than anything, I just wanted to be free from everything that was holding me back, or rather, everything I was using to hold myself back.

With this new vision and courage, I made a few choices I never made before. I decided to turn myself in to the police station because, at this time, I had a warrant for my arrest (again). Because of my honesty, they were willing to work with me, which came as a shocker to me! I also moved into a motel near where my son lived because I couldn't stand to live where I was anymore. The relationship between my son's mother and me got so bad that I needed to take space away. I was using my grandmother's car for a food delivery job. Finally, I decided to tackle my substance use. This was one of the hardest decisions I had ever made. I wasn't able to do it by myself, because every time I was on the brink of being done, I took a wrong turn and decided to do it again. I was at my wit's end, I couldn't figure out what to do, until one moment, when I no longer was allowed to use Grandma's car, I had no more days left in the motel before I had to leave, and I was totally broke, something happened. I prayed again. I asked the universe what I was supposed to do because I had exhausted all of my options. At that moment, I heard the answer loud and clear. I instantly remembered that there was an Alcoholics Anonymous meeting nearby that would be starting in 30 minutes. This was the first time I had heard guidance from my intuition and instantly knew what I was supposed to do if I wanted to make the change I desired. Without thinking, I ran to my grandmother's house, thank god she lived so close, so I could use her car one more time to go to this meeting. I sat through the meeting, and when it was over, I stood up crying and asking the people there for help. A few of the guys my age came to talk with me, and they took me out to eat after the meeting. This is when I first heard of the rehabilitation center I would be going into just 5 days later. Primary Purpose, in Sheffield, Ohio, is where I felt guided to go to get help for my drug use and to have a place to stay while my mind, body, and spirit were being restored to their natural state.

While at Primary Purpose, I really got to work building up my new identity. I went through the 12 steps of Alcoholics Anonymous, took an Intensive Outpatient therapy group, and let some people love me while I figured out how to love myself. I also said my "choices" every morning and every night. After about 75 days in the halfway portion of the facility, completing the program, and getting a job, I was eligible to move up to the ¾ way living area. Now I was living in an apartment-style house with a few other guys who were doing the same thing. I paid rent, went to work, and went to AA meetings. Now that I was in the right head space and earning my own money, I was finally ready to retake "Create Your Destiny" and take the next set of classes. This period of my life had led to some massive changes, and now I was ready to take my new identity and my new skills of reality creation to the next level. Quickly, I started attracting new opportunities in my life, from promotions at work to being asked to lead retreats for Alcoholics Anonymous, and being asked to be a co-author in this book!

These changes were occurring rapidly because of my new outlook on life and the tools I was given. I had developed these spiritual tools that allowed me to tap into my creativity and intuition like never before. I also learned how to listen to my own heart as a guide rather than listening to the advice of people who were not on the same path, nor had the same vision as me. It became abundantly clear to me where I had gone wrong for all of these years. I was programmed to think I should be a certain way, which went against the calling of my heart and soul. In my mind, I held beliefs that did not serve my highest good nor did these beliefs align with what I truly wanted to create in the world. If before I was fighting to travel upstream, now I am flowing with the current, on the path of least resistance. Now, I am focusing on the things I truly love, not what I was taught to value. By changing my focus, I started changing the world around me. By changing the world around me to fit what I feel inside, I've created a perpetual spiral towards creating what I love and loving what I create, leading to more and more joy in my life.

After some time living in the treatment facility, I got to a point where I was ready to move out and move on with my life. I wanted more freedom and less supervision. I had a sponsor with Alcoholics Anonymous at the time, and I noticed that this was another individual who I started to allow in my life and direct the way I was thinking and because I was looking for more creative freedom, I decided to leave the program and facility to explore. This was a very scary moment for me because it meant that I was going to be doing this on my own. At this point, I had no one to mentor me, and I was living off the fly of my own creative desire and intuition. I quickly learned that this was an invitation to free fall into the universe and see if I could manifest my desired reality. After living in my car for a couple of months and spending the rest of my earnings from my previous job, I crash-landed at my grandma's house, and the story continues, however I will it. This is when I learned that having a coach, or someone to hold you accountable for your creations was without a doubt one of the most important aspects of living in a creative orientation. It's imperative to continue in your forward momentum if you desire to keep climbing higher. What I mean by this is, we must build freedom in our lives. If I do nothing and think that I am free, I will not get very far. To create a life that I desire, I must build it, through my actions, creating a character or a version of myself that has already accomplished what I would love to accomplish. By committing to daily habits that build this character and taking aligned, inspired action, I can create the life of my dreams quicker than I thought was possible otherwise.

Today, I live by intuitive means. I love creating YouTube videos and courses helping people understand this work at a deeper level. My intuition helps me discover what my heart really wants to express and I allow myself space to feel how I want and flow into what I desire to create. I am still learning and growing in my process and as long as I am willing to make mistakes, or miss the mark, then I will be more apt to commit myself to the process, focusing on my true end result and creating what I love. Sometimes I make mistakes in my creative process, but I use it to my advantage to learn and grow from. Allowing myself to learn from mistakes and continue to grow and get better, stronger, and more accurate for next time; I will continue to strive, be joyful, and create the things that I truly love in this world.

Freeing myself from the chains of my old mindset, addictions, generational thought patterns, and behaviors has been one of the most impactful things in my life. I'm very grateful for the classes and opportunities I've had in life to learn about these spiritual tools and lessons that allow me to grow better each day. I continually strive to get more free and create more beautiful things in my life so that I can be of service to the next person who is stuck and help them unchain themselves. Impacting one heart has a ripple effect on other hearts, and as we love ourselves and those around us, we are creating more and more love on the planet, creating a better humanity for all.

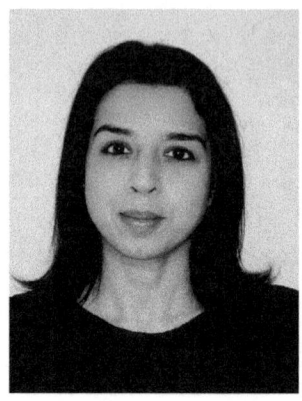

Soniya Barard

Author

https://www.facebook.com/Soniya.Barard

Soniya Barard was born and raised in the heart of the east-end of London, United Kingdom, in the 1980's. This is where she first fell deeply in love with the world.

She enjoyed her time at school and continues to be a life-long student. Maths was her weakest subject, until the arrival of her son, Leo, who taught her the art of mathematics and so much else beyond.

Her work continues to share her art, wisdom and love with those around her who would happily receive it. Her current projects consist of writing, performing, public speaking and community leadership. She seeks to work with all aligned with her mission and purpose.

She can be found embracing her humanity and divinity, in communities and networks around the world.

Something Beyond

By Soniya Barard

There was nothing to be done. Everything was dead. Least of all my heart, but the enemy stood at the gates and surrounded from all sides. There was no escape. Nowhere to escape to. I was a hostage in my mind, in my life, in every direction I turned to look. And I was alone.

It could go so many ways – this thing I called my life, but I was trapped within a torturous puzzle of pain. Confusion reigned supreme, in my own life and it appeared to me, in the lives of others around me, also.

Yes, people were living all around me, going about their days and self-created purposes with more or less rigour. It was often the complete strangers I met that held the most significant presence and grace for me. I could shy away from the truth of who I was in my life, with my family and friends, but there were instances, where all I attempted to grasp of my man-made self fled, and I'd be left naked and vulnerable with somebody also willing to do the same. Sometimes, for only a few brief moments. Sometimes longer. But always, that connection, raw, untamed, free, reaffirmed a sacred truth to me – I am more. More than I know. More than I've done. More than I've been led to believe, or have accepted. There is just so much more to us all. But where does it fit in the real world? How does it fit?

I stood before the confusion of my ever-growing dissatisfaction with the world, others and myself, seeking to reunite the aspects of myself I had so clearly denied or lost the ability to master.

I knew the great ones had existed. Throughout time, they had come into the world delivering awe-inspiring and unique facets of human brilliance, skill and inspiration, often in multifaceted ways. Yet, my world stage was not dominated by such awe and inspiration. No. Something had gone wrong. There was something missing.

Something so fundamental, it seemed to me, that we were operating daily as fragmented parts of our whole selves. In truth, we are always that which we are. Yet, something more is often beckoning our heed and call.

I began my corporate career in engineering and construction in Central London, UK, in my early twenties around 2008, with massive dreams, ambitions and hopes. There was some freedom in my specialist field – information management. It was a brand-spanking new industry borne on the back of the ever-growing demand for accurate, reliable information and data in fast-paced, changing and critical environments.

I loved the buzz of creation and the thrill of project management and coordination. I loved taking care of those I found myself surrounded with. Especially with tea and biscuits. Sometimes, sweets and cakes also.

I often found myself in male-dominated working environments – construction, security and investment banking, to name a few. In some ways, this gave me the grace to define myself to these men directly. I represented much to them that they were unfamiliar with – my age, colour, gender and societal background, not usually found where we happened to be.

This afforded me an outrageous audaciousness in setting my boundaries with others. I discarded the could/would/should – and dealt with people as I found them to be. And sometimes it turned ugly, as all real human interactions have the potential to do. Despite our best intentions and ideas – we're just not able to be everything to everybody all of the time. Sometimes, it gets ugly.

But there were many beautiful moments of growth and connection, warmth and combined spiritual reverence. I love the spiritual conversations more than anything. I have always been this way. I love God, the Almighty, the absolute. I consider Him (out of habit – a bad one at that) omnipresent, omnipotent, omniscient. Gratefully, I was born into a modern-day faith, Sikhism, which taught me gender (and all other types of) equality.

My personal spiritual journey was also heavily influenced by Christianity, the major faith of the country I grew up in, the UK. I call God, Waheguru (Greater Guru) but my saviour, Jesus. The love, all of the love, I accept it wherever I find it.

Love is, for me, God. And what Jesus did for us as a humanity is worthy of infinite praise and admiration.

I adored the Christian hymns and stories and though the scopes of both my childhood religions varied – there was significant overlap in context. I found them to be complementary rather than at odds with one another (at their inner depths) – as I found many other religions, faiths, ideologies, etc. to also be.

And so my spirituality was strongly tied to the structures around me until I developed the confidence and faith to also contribute to the creation of such structures.

To be honest, to simultaneously grasp two ideologies/world faiths at once (or let's be real – even in succession) was considered, when I was growing up, absolute bad taste, desecration and foul. To be avoided at all costs. By everyone, including the religious institutions themselves. To proclaim no faith at birth – risky. Outcast. To proclaim no faith as absolute – incriminating. The opponents are forever ready to battle. No one lets anyone else ahead at the risk of being left behind or led astray. It's survival of the fittest we're told, but do we know the power and glory that our creator bestowed upon us? Do we really believe it? Truly?

I do. I believe in the eternal longing of my soul and the peace it affords me in a sometimes chaotic and harsh world environment. I believe in a multidimensional universe of infinite potential, forever within reach and grasp for my consideration, employment and enjoyment. I am a child of God. A lover. A poet. A muse.

I believe. But I find I'm often the only one or in the minority. And so, I shut down and hold on.

There are things in this world and life more precious and significant to us than all else. I call these my priorities and values. They aren't all tangible. There are many significant intangible aspects to our lives. We simply comprehend our lives and ourselves the best we can, at any given moment. This is the best I expect from myself and others. To be the best we can be – in full spectacular God-given glory and power. To do better, as we realise better, to always strive towards better.

Perhaps this is how I became so engrossed in concepts of evolution, theoretical sciences and ascension – the seemingly mystical laws and veils beyond our usual sense of perception. Not only was the existence of such planes of multidimensional reality so self-evident once presented, but it really opened up the universe to each and every individual to co-create and magically and authentically inhabit.

The desire to realise such a world within my lifetime led me to commit my life to the pursuit and harbouring of it. A brave new world. But no one felt brave, sure or sane. Not for long anyway. I was in my mid-twenties and I knew the time for me to grow up had come. I had to take responsibility – and I currently had two – myself and my family, biological and all.

My cosmic identity was always so self-evident to me. I was a child of the cosmos – literally and physically. The universe as we comprehend it, always stood to me to be our closest approximation of understanding the divine and greater beyond. Whether you looked at it scientifically or spiritually – it all worked out the same.

I understood the reasons why we found ourselves in a spiritual conundrum individually and collectively. Our history of rape, pillaging and conquest clearly documented in records across time had led to the destruction and downfall of certain critical aspects of self, and the previously collectively held self-knowledge.

We were all as lost as each other and though there were those who had achieved spiritual attainment and knowledge – they were held by the strict laws and codes that protected their faith as an identity.

I was alone. Because I chose to be. I didn't want to attain my God-given rights and powers secretly, hidden away from the eager heart and hungry soul. I saw the desperation in the eyes of those around me – in flashes and in rampages – I saw myself in all. God in all. Yearning to be free in a world that had shut down and devalued the essentials of life. And here we were, dying in our masses, physically, emotionally, mentally, spiritually, in each and every way that we could be truly alive, we were also dying.

And I yearned to be free. Now and here in this world I found myself in. Not in some distant future or undefined dream.

Heaven and hell are both here and now within the world – anything beyond is an individual's own journey and reconciliation to be found. I chose heaven over hell. I chose freedom over secrecy. I chose the ultimate dream – heaven on Earth, for all of humanity.

Arguments against dreams often relate to the impossibility or improbability of such large-scale visions. I did not give a fuck. I did not care how ridiculous I seemed or sounded. All else was death to me. I needed God like I needed my breath. And I chose to serve His will, to dedicate myself to both love (God) and truth (his "name") in each and every way that I could truly grasp. This became my ultimate faith, goal and purpose. To become a living temple, a vessel of the holy and divine. To tend the living spark that connects me to my ultimate creator.

This I knew to be my divinely gifted birthright. God knew the reasons why. God's plan. God's way. God's timing. I was set and ready to begin, and to make my mark.

I found myself alone, in a home, community and country largely occupied with "fancier" concerns. Material needs and wants. The absence of which is always so clear to see and sense. I did not begrudge anyone their daily bread, bed or even beer. The deficiencies within humanity as a whole affect us all differently. We're all doing the best we can, in a sometimes inhumane, cruel and nasty world.

Sometimes, it gets nonsensical. Beyond that which you comprehend, you can imagine. Sometimes this knowledge is all the power you need. The power of imagination.

It isn't meant to always be a certain way, there is no guiding map for humanity, and should the way ahead be led, it should be led by us all collectively, as best as we can envisage and relate to the masses at large.

This was evident to me, yet the way forward on my own path to power, was to claim every victory I could, individually and collectively, as well as deal with the consistent failures and struggles that we all constantly face and fear. I was alone, but I will never be outside the collective. In this way, I was able to exist, singularly (as far as is actually possible) and as part of a greater whole.

It was my journey alone, to choose and take, but the repercussions and representations I made, were not mine alone.

Patents are such strange things to me. Copyright and intellectual property rights – it's a con, really. It's all good and well to acknowledge and reward achievement and progress – vital to ensure consistency, quality and adherence as necessary. But to take from the public what is rightfully also collectively theirs – and to make it completely inaccessible to them without any recourse (or limited recourse) to continue the good work ... seems insane to me. We pay so many times, in so many ways, for things that ultimately belong to us. Make it make sense.

Individually, my rights are more limited, tarred and tainted by the armour we all carry to preserve our dignity and God-given grace. Strengths and weaknesses, we all have them – though the shape and size of the doorway through to them vary continuously.

Collectively, I am stronger. Tarred, tainted, armoured, still. But with access and inspiration from the endless strengths and weaknesses we collectively hold.

The doorways. Oh, the doorways we hold both individually and thus also collectively. Portals to other worlds. The Earth itself is so demonstrably a collection of worlds within worlds.

We've lost control. Nearly everything is wrong. We've advanced as a modern technological age and yet so many of us fundamentally struggle to provide the basics for ourselves and our loved ones. It's possible, yes, but it shouldn't be this bloody hard. We're tired. We're dying. And yet the embers of our dying flames stand ready to ignite always. We've held.

When people talk about seeds and fruits of the spirit, I always imagine it to look something like this. To carry seeds is to carry the spark of something that has ignited your soul's passion but has not yet come to fruition. Try as we might to forget, they burn like flames in our spirit forever guiding us towards our greater destiny.

In this lifetime, or not. In this dimension, or not. At any given opportunity – the seeds ripen and grow and eventually blossom and bloom.

This is the growth I advocate for and seek to nurture, both simultaneously within my own soul, for where else do I really hold my power, and within the world at large, in the roles and responsibilities I commit to, and in the demonstration of my own humanity and self-empowerment. This to me is real self-mastery and the only battle really worth fighting. The battle within.

There is much to be said and explored about consciousness. Ultimately, we understand the universe to be mental, a living mind, to which we contribute with our own. Old-view scientific models (they removed ether officially from the Western modern sciences in the early 1900s) complement this world perspective.

The reasons for coming away from such an approach were at first a grand mystery to me. Why did we turn away from a more unified yet multidimensional approach to living? When I studied the fundamental sciences at university, the little we knew and the much we left out (or had lost access to knowing) was clear and loud to me. There was still much to be discovered and established.

I remember being taught in one of my first science lessons at secondary school, that electricity was a flow of electrons. Nice, but I had to ask – okay, but what is it really? My dear, dedicated teacher had no response, beyond that. A flow of electrons. Evidently, there's still much more to be discovered and established.

It turns out, we're good at getting ahead without any real idea of where we're getting ahead to. Shock. Awe. Gasp. With great power comes great responsibility and when none can bear it, that power effectively dies or lays dormant, until it can be carried or incarnated as a real living power again.

I once feared that all lasting hope had been lost. Previous knowledge once collectively held, gone. Humanity degraded and doomed.

But through coming across mentors and like-minded individuals globally – I finally understood that nothing could be lost, for we remained created in the image of the creator, with infinite potential, capabilities and power. This right, gifted to us from beyond, extends beyond. It's so naturally obvious, where one is open to it.

So, I set out to create my part towards a greater good, a greater whole. A better world, for myself and those depending on me first and foremost, and also for those around me in need and want, as I was gifted the opportunity to do so.

There were many magical journeys that followed and my world expanded exponentially within a short time. I was not alone in my quest, allies from near and far, past, present and future, came to present themselves and offer aligned service.

To know I was not alone was enough for me. Truly, I've always known I've not yet been alone in this life. But to have a tangible support network was incredible and invaluable. To be held. Seen. Truly. Critiqued and appreciated, in genuine heartfelt service to the individual and greater good. This was the education I had been seeking my whole life. The education of intuition, genius, creativity and self-mastery.

My doors were flying open. The world started discussing a global ascension event. What a perfect avenue for bringing in the kingdom of heaven, I mused. Even if we fell short, any growth or evolution could be life-altering for everyone.

I volunteered, as I always do, on the follow-through of my heart's pull. Whatever aligned with my true nature and purpose, I took on board. Whatever did not, I let go. Often, it was a partial exchange. Such is the nature of "truth".

Truth can be considered objective or subjective. There is very little (if anything) we can claim as objectively true. Almost anything can also be subjectively true. This first and essential premise when dealing with any form of "truth" guides us to realise the nature of God and the universe. We ultimately find connection, correspondence and our true creativity by building our own truth.

Now whether you believe in God or not, it is totally non-dictatory to the matter. Even those who are able to grasp such a concept as God, rarely, truly find and enter the domain of their lord. God doesn't ask to be found or believed in anyway. God asks we follow their will & command, to basically love God, yourself & others. We all meet at the appointed time and hour.

I understand God to be love, and his/her name to be truth. I believe Jesus died for my sins and gifted us everlasting, eternal life in the kingdom of his father's heaven. I believe in the fruits of the spirit – blazing as fires of divinely inspired creation. Very little is objectively true, yet truth exists, unchanged, unchanging, infinitely evident. The truth needs no defence. It just is.

So with this newly established information and experience, I found myself outgrown to much of what I thought I was and had created for myself. I yearned to break free of my self-constructed limits and constraints.

In my mind, I had conquered my field and city upon the "real" world once I worked in collaboration with the government and was told, perhaps rather innocently, that they needed a "me" (they referred to my role as information manager, but wow, what an honour)!

I found my successes lived deep within me, though there were many superficial ones. Does anyone else really care what we get up to? No. Do I really care? Well, I better, or else, what is the point of reaching a goal no one truly, really cares about? I realised pretty quickly – people like you to be well, but what that actually means, takes or looks like, is anybody else's guess and best approximation. They simply know you to be well – because you express it to be so.

Success and failure carry us through to the land of the living, to the real material world that is accessible to us. Sometimes it is only by creating something, by experiencing it directly, that we truly assimilate what we are yearning from that experience. Sometimes it lasts. It seeds and spreads and shoots for the sky. Sometimes it does not. Sometimes, the lesson is what we do not desire, but ultimately, this again redirects us back to our truth with greater awareness and compassion, for ourselves and others.

There is no way it has to be, no one way it is. And so, I left my comfortable UK life, to seek greater opportunities and avenues in faraway lands.

I found native tribespeople and shamans to be most particularly interesting. The knowledge and wisdom carried through the ages still exists in select communities, a treasure still waiting to be largely acknowledged and appreciated by humanity as a collective whole.

Eventually, I found myself living in and amongst such a wise society. Eventually, all that was not really, truly aligned with my spirit and spirit-led purposes dissipated.

Life became beautiful. Truly. Magnificently. Not on the basis of any external criteria, but through the determined and focused alignment of my heart, mind, body and soul. I started to exist from my whole being and the world started to respond with the same energy. Everything became alive, at long last. I was truly alive.

There were falls, crashes and challenges ahead, I knew, but this thing I had finally discovered, this self-identity I had finally encompassed, could go nowhere. It was me. And I had finally seen, acknowledged and accepted myself.

I was the treasure I was seeking, or the avenue to it in any case. All else became obsolete without the participation of my soul/spirit.

There was nothing to be done, except to continue with the path I was on. My gifts so clearly divine in nature, reunited with its source. Once, twice, many times, through many divine experiences. I was led on a divine path.

As divine purposes go, they are completely optional, as far as free will is concerned. Divine will is something beyond, a collaborative effort of sorts. There is no sway in the will of the divine, but of course, there is a relationship with and to it, if you so choose it to be.

The sword of truth, they say, is held by the mighty and worthy. And obviously, they have to be willing, too.

One might look at these words – mighty, worthy, willing and try to assess their true definition. One might look at all words and do the same.

Confusion reigns supreme. But hark, the herald angels sing, glory to the newborn king.

Whatever plans the divine sets forth for me, I willingly embrace with my open loving tender heart. Love leads. Love guides. Love always wins.

If I had a part to play in our collective and cosmic ascension – I played it. Not perfectly. Hell, no. But wholly, truly, really, I did. And if I'm to truly herald the breaking of a new day, a new world for us all, I must release the need to know exactly what that will look like. For it is not in my hands alone.

The transformation must begin from within. This is no throwaway slogan. It all begins and ends with us.

The foundations and structures we build upon, determine the end result. I pray we begin at the beginning, which would be where we are collectively today, what works, and what so evidently does not.

Conflict is a tool for greater self-awareness. We must be responsible in our approach and mature in our actions. Boundaries are key.

Love, I came to realise, exists in almost everyone and everything. We hold great significance over who we pair or mate with. Yet, the most significant bonds to me, transcend all real choices. There is a pull. There already exists a connection. We just happen to find it. Or not, as the case may be.

The longing of my loins led me to realise the inextricable and constant bond of family. Genetic, biological, and spiritual, it continues on. I realised the closest bond I could ever foster was that with my children, my parents, with that which I came from, and to that which I continue with. This is the starkest reality for me as a woman in today's world.

The longing, oh, the constant longing of my heart, is an extension of the love I share and carry across multiple planes and dimensions of existence. These are my gifts and heritage to share, should I so choose to.

Join the movement, share your story!

#AsIfByMagic

We hope the stories you've read in this book have inspired you to trust in your inner guidance, follow your heart and start (or continue) living intuitively. The authors of this book come from different walks of life and have shared their personal journeys of breaking free from the logic-driven, societal expectations that keep people from having a full experience of life. They've chosen to trust their hearts, and as a result, they've created lives that are nothing short of magical.

But this book is just the beginning.

The world is full of people who, like you, are seeking the courage to follow their hearts and live in alignment with their true selves. If you've felt a spark of inspiration reading these stories, we invite you to take the next step.

It's time to add your story to this movement. Whether you've already started your own intuitive journey or you're just beginning to explore the possibilities, there's a place for you in the As If By Magic community. This is a space for individuals who are willing to take the road less travelled, to embrace the unknown, follow their hearts and to trust in the unseen forces that guide them towards living their true potential.

We believe that every story has the power to inspire, and that's why we're inviting you to share yours with the world. You may be on the edge of a breakthrough, about to embark on a journey that will change everything for you, or you may already have the experience and insights that could guide others. Whatever stage you're at, your story matters.

Here's how you can get involved:

- **Share Your Story**: We want to hear from you! Join the conversation and share how intuitive living has impacted your life. Share your personal story, your challenges, your breakthroughs, or your dreams, and use the hashtag **#AsIfByMagic** on social media to join a global network of people living in alignment with their intuition. Whether your journey is just beginning, or you've already experienced profound transformations, your story has the potential to inspire others to take their own bold steps.

- **Join the As If By Magic Community**: Head over to www.asifbymagic.com.au to become part of a growing community of like-minded individuals. Here, you'll find a wealth of resources, including exclusive content, workshops, and ongoing support to help you on your journey. The more people we have sharing their stories, the more powerful this movement will become. Together, we can create a world where intuitive living is no longer the exception but the norm.

- **Get Inspired and Empowered**: By joining the community, you're not only embracing your own potential but you're also contributing to a collective shift in how we all live our lives. You'll find inspiration, tools, and connections to continue your personal journey and to make an even greater impact in the world around you. Every story shared, every heart opened, and every soul awakened contributes to the magic that is unfolding in our world.

Living intuitively isn't about following the crowd or waiting for permission. It's about daring to go against the grain, trusting your heart, and stepping into the unknown with the courage to create a life that is uniquely yours.

This is the essence of **As If By Magic**.

Are you ready to take the next step? Your story could be the one that sparks someone else's transformation. You're not alone on this journey, and there's no better time than now to share your truth, inspire others, and grow alongside an empowered community of people who are committed to living from the heart.

Let's keep the magic alive—**join the movement today.**

Visit www.asifbymagic.com.au to learn about sharing your story.

Together we can create a community inspiring others to follow their hearts, trust their intuition, and allow transformation to unfold effortlessly—**AS IF BY MAGIC**